NOVEL STRATEGIES IN LYMPHEDEMA

Edited by **Alberto Vannelli**

Novel Strategies in Lymphedema
Edited by Alberto Vannelli

Published by InTech
Janeza Trdine 9, 51000 Rijeka, Croatia

Publishing Process Manager Maja Bozicevic

Technical Editor Teodora Smiljanic

Cover Designer InTech Design Team

Additional hard copies can be obtained from orders@intechopen.com

Novel Strategies in Lymphedema, Edited by Alberto Vannelli
p. cm.
978-953-307-929-5

Meet the editor

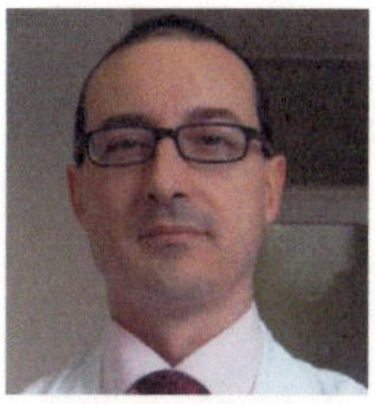

Dr Alberto Vannelli, MD, is a lecturer in Oncological Lymphology at Università degli Studi of Milan, Italy. He received his university degree with a dissertation on "Assisted circulation by extracorporeal bypass techniques in liver transplantation", and his specialization in General Surgery with a dissertation on "Conservative surgery in rectal cancer". He received both degrees from the University of Milan, Italy. From 2001 he was an attending physician in Colorectal Division at Fondazione IRCCS Istituto Nazionale dei Tumori of Milan, Italy. Vannelli first became interested in the lymphatic circulation and began seminal studies on the pathophysiology of lymphadenectomy, pelvic lymphedema and pelvic surgery. Since 2011 he has been a consultant surgeon in the General Surgery Division at Valduce Hospital in Como, Italy.

Contents

Introductory Chapter

A Brief Overview of Lymphology: Past, Present and Future

Alberto Vannelli
Foundation IRCCS "National Institute of Cancer", Milan
Faculty Lecturer in lymphology, University of the Study of Milan, Italy

1. Introduction

The human body has two circulatory systems. These are the cardiovascular system and the lymphatic system. They are part of the immune system comprising a network of conduits called lymphatic vessels that carry a clear fluid called lymph (from Latin lympha "water") towards the heart. There are many milestones in the history of the lymphatic system. The lymphoid system can be broadly divided into the conducting system and the lymphoid tissue. The conducting system carries the lymph and consists of tubular vessels that include the lymph capillaries, the lymph vessels, and the right and left thoracic ducts. The lymphoid tissue is primarily involved in immune responses and consists of lymphocytes and other white blood cells enmeshed in connective tissue through which the lymph passes. Regions of the lymphoid tissue that are densely packed with lymphocytes are known as lymphoid follicles. Lymphoid tissue can either be structurally well organized as lymph nodes or may consist of loosely organized lymphoid follicles known as the mucosa-associated lymphoid tissue (MALT). Lymph vessels called lacteals are present in the lining of the gastrointestinal tract, predominantly in the small intestine. While most other nutrients absorbed by the small intestine are passed on to the portal venous system to drain via the portal vein into the liver for processing, fats (lipids) are passed on to the lymphatic system to be transported to the blood circulation via the thoracic duct. (There are exceptions, for example medium-chain triglycerides are fatty acid esters of glycerol that passively diffuse from the gastrointestinal tract to the portal system.) The enriched lymph originating in the lymphatics of the small intestine is called chyle. As the blood circulates, fluid leaks out into the body tissues. This fluid is important because it carries food to the cells and waste back to the bloodstream. The nutrients that are released to the circulatory system are processed by the liver, having passed through the systemic circulation. The lymph system is a one-way system, transporting interstitial fluid back to blood. Lymphatics were discovered by chance, but were misunderstood for a very long time. Up to the early twentieth century the accurate description of lymphatics was deemed necessary to promote advances in oncology (Rouviere, 1932). The study of lymphatic drainage of various organs is important in diagnosis, prognosis, and treatment of cancer. The lymphatic system, because of its physical proximity to many tissues of the body, is responsible for carrying cancerous cells between the various parts of the body in a process called metastasis. The intervening lymph nodes can trap the cancer cells. If they are not successful in destroying the cancer cells the nodes may become sites of secondary tumours. As editor of this book it is my intention in this brief introductory chapter to provide a sampling of some of the varied topics related to the discipline of lymphology. Whetting the readers' appetite for this subject will enable them to better enjoy the many superb multi-authored chapters written with an international perspective that follow.

2. Past

Hippocrates was one of the first people to mention the lymphatic system in the 5th century BC. In his work "On Joints," he briefly mentioned the lymph nodes in one sentence. Rufus of Ephesus, a Roman physician, identified the axillary, inguinal and mesenteric lymph nodes as well as the thymus during the 1st to 2nd century AD (Ambrose, 2006).

Erasistrate, the most famous Alexandrian anatomist, observed lymph vessels in animals, but he mistook them for arteries. Another anatomist, Herophile mistook them for veins. However, the latter also referred to "glandular bodies", which must be regarded as the current lymph nodes. The first mention of lymphatic vessels was in 3rd century BC by Herophilos, a Greek anatomist living in Alexandria, who incorrectly concluded that the "absorptive veins of the lymphatics", by which he meant the lacteals (lymph vessels of the intestines), drained into the hepatic portal veins, and thus into the liver (Ambrose, 2006). Findings of Ruphus and Herophilos were further propagated by the Greek physician Galen, who described the lacteals and mesenteric lymph nodes which he observed in his dissection of apes and pigs in the 2nd century AD. Until the 17th century, ideas of Galen were most prevalent. Accordingly, it was believed that the blood was produced by the liver from chyle contaminated with ailments by the intestine and stomach, to which various spirits were added by other organs, and that this blood was consumed by all the organs of the body.

This theory required that the blood be consumed and produced many times over. His ideas remained unchallenged until the 17th century, and even then were defended by some physicians (Fanous et al, 2007). In the 16th century, Nicolas Massa briefly described some lymph vessels of the human kidneys (1536), and Bartolomeo Eustachi (1564) made the first accurate description of the thoracic duct in a horse, which he called "Vena alba thoracis". Eustachi only observed its thoracic course and its connection with the subclavian or internal jugular vein. In the 17th century, many famous European anatomists such as Gaspare Aselli, Thomas Bartholin, Olof Rudbeck, Jean Pecquet and Frederik Ruysch made important contributions to the knowledge of the lymphatic system (Arvy & Rivet, 1976).

The Italian surgeon Gaspare Aselli was a pupil of his famous compatriot Gabriele Falloppio. In 1622, he discovered the lacteal vessels while displaying the abdominal viscera of a dog at an anatomical demonstration. As it happened, the animal had been fed shortly before the dissection, and Aselli could therefore observe milky "fibers" running on the mesentery. He first mistook them for nerves and decided to cut them in the course of his demonstration. He then observed a whitish liquid flowing out of these "fibers" and came to the conclusion that they were vessels. Some days later, he began to verify his observations in other animal species: cats, lambs, cows, pigs, and even a horse he bought only for this purpose (Regis & Kaoru, 1971). Unfortunately, before his death in 1626, Aselli could not confirm the existence of lacteal vessels in humans. Aselli's book was published posthumously under the editorship of Alessandro Tadini and Luigi Settala (1627). The Danish anatomists Thomas

Bartholin (1616-1680) and Olof Rudbeck (1630-1702) published numerous studies on lymphatics and disagreed over their distribution (Hagelin, 1989). Jean Pecquet (1622-1681) described the confluence of abdominal lymph trunks and the cysterna chyli at the origin of the thoracic duct in a dog (Pecquet, 1651). Eleven years later, Frederik Ruysch (1638-1731) established the existence of valves in the lymphatic vessels. He presented this in a small book dedicated to his three much-admired teachers, Franciscus De Le Boe, Johann van Home and Florentius Schuyl (Ruysch, 1665; Luyendijk-Elshout, 1964).

The Italian anatomist Paolo Mascagni (1755-1815) studied at Siena under Pietro Tabarrini (1702-1780). His most successful research was on lymphatics, and led first to the submission of preliminary results in 1784, in respect of which the French Academy of Sciences awarded a prize, and second, to the publication of one of the most striking atlases in 1787. By using a very simple method (a tubular needle bent at right angle), he was able to discover about fifty per cent of all the lymphatic vessels now known (Norman, 1978). Moreover, he established that every lymph vessel must in its course enter at least one lymph node; disproved the existence of arterial and venous lymph vessels, and concluded that the lymphatic system originates from all the cavities and surfaces of the body.

Mascagni's procedure for the injection of superficial lymph vessels was widely used in the following century. In order to avoid filling the deep lymph vessels during the injection of the superficial ones, Mascagni recommended injecting glue in the arteries first, then cooling the specimen. In this way, all lymph vessels (superficial and deep) became collapsed. For the selective injection of the superficial vessels, he warmed up the surface of the specimen so that the glue could soften, therefore making the superficial lymph vessels permeable again.

Ernest Alexandre Lauth (1803-1837) belonged to a famous Strasbourg family of anatomists. He studied under Vincent Fohmann (1794-1837), and carried out researches on the lymph system in birds (1825) and people (1824, 1829). In his 1829 handbook, he gives a detailed account of the injection and preparation of lymph vessels, which may be summarized as follows: the choice of the body to be prepared is very important. It should be young, robust, and should preferably have died of an acute episode.

If the body is fat, lymph vessels will be difficult to identify and Lauth recommends arterial injection with lukewarm water, so that the tissues become infiltrated. Another procedure is to inject arteries and veins with wax and to let the specimen soak for some days. The development of gas in the lymph vessels will then make them more visible, and the previous injection of wax allows an easy differentiation from arterial and venous vessels. This is the way the English anatomist William Cruikshank discovered the lymph vessels of the heart and the uterus in 1786.

Finally, Lauth reminds us that hypertrophied organs make the dissection of lymph vessels easier. According to Lauth, the lymph vessels of a gravid uterus are thicker in diameter than the feather of a crow. In the nineteenth century, the lymph vessels were usually injected with mercury. Lauth stresses the fact that mercury must be as pure as possible, and must in any case be filtered through a piece of chamois leather. To check the purity of the mercury, he put a drop of mercury on an inclined plate. If the drop slid without dirtying the plate, the mercury was pure enough for the injection. If not, it meant it contained traces of lead or tin and could not be used for anatomical preparations. However, other products could also be used. For the injection of thick lymph vessels (thoracic duct or right lymphatic duct), Lauth writes that plaster yields good results provided one takes care of the orientation of the valves. In addition, he reminds us that his colleague Andre Marie Constant Dumeril made successful injections of lymph vessels with milk, provided the specimen was not intended to be preserved by drying. Other anatomists injected black ink by blowing into a tube connected to a thin glass needle. This procedure was used for the first study of lymphatics in Japan (Husiya & Waran, 1805). To inject mercury into the superficial lymph vessels, Lauth carefully removed a small square of skin, located a vessel, made a small incision in its wall with a lancet, and introduced a thin glass or steel tube into the vessel. Owing to the high number of anastomoses, three injections are sufficient to inject all superficial lymph vessels of the lower limb: one injection on the hallux, a second on the fifth toe, and a third one behind the medial malleolus. For the same reason, three or four injections in various parts of the hand will fill all superficial lymph vessels of the upper limb (here he is at variance with Mascagni, who wrote that at least twenty injections are necessary for a whole limb).

Marie Philibert Constant Sappey was a French anatomist born in Cernon, near the city of Bourg-en-Bresse. He conducted numerous studies on the lymphatic system up to the middle of the 19th century. In the second edition of his treatise on anatomy in 1869, he gives a summary of the important points that have to be taken into consideration for a successful injection of the lymphatics. Sappey differs with Lauth regarding the choice of body. Sappey recommends the body of man who died of a chronic disease because it will be sufficiently emaciated. The body of a child should only be used to study the lymphatics of the head, the tongue, the soft palate, the gums or the scrotum. Regardless of the specimen, however, Sappey thought that the injection of lymphatics should always be carried out in summer because a high temperature makes the progression of mercury easier.

3. Present

In today's world the interest in lymphology can be considered extraordinary, even in view of the increasing incidence of lymphedema, and covering all ages and lymphatic malformations, troncular and extra-troncular. Several national scientific societies, associations and study groups, which fall within the guidelines of the International Society of Lymphology and the International Union of Phlebology, are contributing to the awareness of these problems and to their solutions, which the international scientific community has already been studying for a long time. The study and the management of the lymphatic diseases requires the co-operation of many specialists such as lymphologists, internists, oncologists, dermatologists, vascular internists, phlebologists, physicians specializing in infective diseases, radiologists, gynecologists, surgeons, vascular surgeons, plastic surgeons, nurses, physiotherapists, gymnastic instructors and diet instructors.

The lymphatic system clears away infection and keeps your body fluids in balance. If it's not working properly, fluid builds in your tissues and causes swelling called lymphedema. Other lymphatic system problems can include infections, blockage, and cancer. Lymphedema results from an alteration of lymphatic vessels as a consequence of malformation (primary) or mechanical damage (secondary) (Warren et al, 2007), consistent with an equal distribution in the upper and lower limbs, neck, scrotum and pubis (Purushotham et al, 2007; Fang et al 2008). It is most frequently seen after lymph node dissection, surgery or radiation therapy, in which damage to the lymphatic system is caused during the treatment of cancer, most notably breast cancer. In many patients with cancer, this condition does not develop until months or even years after the therapy has concluded. Lymphedema may also be associated with accidents or certain diseases or problems that may inhibit the lymphatic system from functioning properly. In tropical areas of the world, a common cause of secondary lymphedema is filariasis, a parasitic infection. It can also be caused by the compromising of the lymphatic system, as a result of cellulitis. While the exact cause of primary lymphedema is still unknown, it generally occurs due to the poorly developed or missing lymph nodes or channels in the body. Lymphedema may be present at birth, develop at the onset of puberty (praecox), or not become apparent for many years into adulthood (tarda). In men, lower-limb primary lymphedema is most common, occurring in one or both legs. Some cases of lymphedema may be associated with other vascular abnormalities. Secondary lymphedema affects both men and women. In women, it is most prevalent in the upper limbs after breast cancer surgery and lymph node dissection, occurring in the arm on the side of the body in which the surgery is performed. Head and neck lymphedema can be caused by surgery or radiation therapy for tongue or throat cancer. It may also occur in the lower limbs or groin after surgery for colon, ovarian or uterine cancer, in which removal of lymph nodes or radiation therapy is required. Surgery or treatment of prostate, colon and testicular cancers may result in secondary lymphedema, particularly when lymph nodes have been removed or damaged. The onset of secondary lymphedema in patients who have had cancer surgery has also been linked to aircraft flight (likely due to decreased cabin pressure). For cancer survivors, therefore, wearing a prescribed and properly fitted compression garment may help decrease swelling during air travel. Some cases of lower-limb lymphedema have been associated with the use of tamoxifen, due to the blood clots and deep vein thrombosis (DVT) that can be caused by this medication. Resolution of the blood clots or DVT is needed before lymphedema treatment can be initiated.

Today the treatment for lymphedema varies depending on the severity of the edema and the degree of fibrosis of the affected limb. Most people with lymphedema follow a daily regimen of treatment as suggested by their physician or certified lymphedema therapist. The most common treatments for lymphedema are a combination of manual compression lymphatic massage, compression garments or bandaging. Complex decongestive physiotherapy is an empiric system of lymphatic massage, skin care, and compressive garments. Although a combination treatment program may be ideal, any of the treatments can be done individually.

Elastic compression garments are worn by people with lymphedema on the affected limb following complete decongestive therapy to maintain edema reduction. Depending on the therapist's discretion, a compression garment may be custom-fitted or purchased in over-the-counter, standard sizes.

Compression garments are meant to be worn every day to maintain edema reduction and must be replaced on a regular basis. Support garments may be the only garment of choice for patients with Scrotal edema.

Compression bandaging, also called wrapping, is the application of several layers of padding and short-stretch bandages to the involved areas. Short-stretch bandages are preferred over long-stretch bandages (such as those normally used to treat sprains) as the long-stretch bandages cannot produce the proper therapeutic tension necessary to safely reduce lymphedema and may in fact end up producing a tourniquet effect. During activity, whether exercise or daily activities, the short-stretch bandages enhance the pumping action of the lymph vessels by providing increased resistance for them to push against. This encourages lymphatic flow and helps to soften fluid-swollen areas.

Compression pump technology utilizes a multi-chambered pneumatic sleeve with overlapping cells to promote movement of lymph fluid. Pump therapy may be used in addition to other treatments such as compression bandaging and manual lymph drainage. In many cases, pump therapy may help soften fibrotic tissue and therefore potentially enable more efficient lymphatic drainage. Sequential pump therapy may also be used as a home treatment method, usually as part of a regimen also involving compression garments or wrapping. A Stanford University medical study showed that patients receiving the combined modalities of complete decongestive therapy or manual lymph drainage (MLD/CDT) and pneumatic pumping had a greater overall reduction in limb volume than patients receiving only MLD/CDT (Szuba et al, 2002). However, some therapists have begun to raise concern that compression pumps can cause genital swelling when used on persons with leg lymphedema.

Complete decongestive therapy (CDT) is a primary tool in lymphedema management consisting of manual manipulation of the lymphatic ducts, short-stretch compression bandaging, therapeutic exercise, and skin care (National Lymphedema Network Medical Advisor Committee, 2011). The technique was pioneered by Emil Vodder in the 1930s for the treatment of chronic sinusitis and other immune disorders. Initially, CDT involves frequent visits to a certified therapist with a doctor's prescription. Once the lymphedema is reduced, increased patient participation is required for ongoing care, along with the use of elastic compression garments and non-elastic directional flow foam garments. Manual manipulation of the lymphatic ducts consists of gentle, rhythmic massaging of the skin to stimulate the flow of lymph and its return to the blood circulation system. In the blood's passage through the kidneys, the excess fluid is filtered out and eliminated from the body through urination. The treatment is very gentle and a typical session will involve drainage of the neck, trunk, and involved extremity (in that order), lasting approximately 40 to 60 minutes. CDT is generally effective on non-fibrotic lymphedema and less effective on more fibrotic legs, although it has been shown to help break up fibrotic tissue.

Surgical techniques for correcting lymphedema may be excisional or physiological. However, surgery for lymphedema does not cure the disease or eliminate the need for decongestive treatment. Surgical treatment is used only in extreme cases in order to reduce the weight of the affected limb, to help minimize the frequency of inflammatory attacks, to improve cosmesis, and to potentially reduce the risk of secondary angiosarcoma (National Lymphedema Network Medical Advisor Committee, 2011). Although surgery has been shown to reduce edema in the short-term, there is a lack of evidence to suggest that it is beneficial in the long-term. Excisional techniques include three steps: first - circumferential excision of the lymphedematous tissue followed by skin grafting (Charles technique), longitudinal removal of the affected segment of skin and subcutaneous tissue and primary closure (Homans technique), excision of subcutaneous tissue and tunneling of a dermal flap through the fascia into a muscular compartment of the leg (Thompson technique); second - lympholymphatic anastomosis (autologous lymphatic grafts to bridge obstructed lymphatic segments), lymphovenous shunt (anastomosis of lymphatic channels to veins), lymphangioplasty enteromesenteric flap omental transfer (pedicled portion of omentum transposed to the affected limb); third - modified liposuction that has been developed in Sweden in recent years to remove adipose tissue associated with longstanding lymphedema, primarily in the upper region. This last technique is meant to reduce the volume of a limb and does not cure lymphedema. Compression garments and compression bandages must still be worn after the operation.

Low-level laser therapy (LLLT) was cleared by the US Food and Drug Administration (FDA) for the treatment of lymphedema in November 2006 (El Segundo, 2006). According to the US National Cancer Institute, studies suggest that low-level laser therapy may be effective in reducing lymphedema in a clinically meaningful way for some women. Two cycles of laser treatment were found to be effective in reducing the volume of the affected arm, extracellular fluid, and tissue hardness in approximately one-third of patients with post-mastectomy lymphedema at three months post-treatment. Suggested rationales for laser therapy include a potential decrease in fibrosis, stimulation of macrophages and the immune system, and a possible role in encouraging lymphangiogenesis (Carati et al, 2003).

4. Future

Lymphedema is a chronic and irreversible disease with significant negative consequences for the patient, as the resulting aesthetic deformities may make it impossible to continue their career and may lead to social isolation. In this book the authors deal with novel strategies in lymphedema. Still today, physicians and surgeons diagnose lymphedema relatively infrequently and the literature relating to the prevalence of lymphedema is limited. However it is correct to assume that in the future there will be an increase in incidence in primary as well as in secondary lymphedema.

Jin-Hong Chang in her chapter, presents lymphangiogenesis as a complex process that involves the interplay of many molecules with redundant mechanisms. The author deals with specific molecules that have shown the most promise as therapeutic targets including the vascular endothelial growth factors (VEGFs) and their receptors (VEGFRs), COX-2 selective inhibitors, tumor necrosis factor (TNF)-α, and transforming growth factor (TGF)-β.

Primary congenital lymphedema (Milroy disease), representing 10 per cent of primary, is present at birth and associated with an autosomal dominant familial history (Dahlberg et al, 1983). Mutations in the FLT4 gene cause some cases of Milroy disease. The FLT4 gene provides instructions for producing a protein called vascular endothelial growth factor receptor 3 (VEGFR-3), which regulates the development and maintenance of the lymphatic system. About 10 to 15 per cent of people with a mutation in the FLT4 gene do not develop the features of Milroy disease. Today, some of the possible treatments for Milroy's disease from various sources may include: exercise and elevation of extremity, elastic stockings, proper skin hygiene, antibiotics, benzathine penicillin, split-thickness skin grafts, and pedicular transfer of skin. Genetic testing is becoming almost practical, defining a limited number of specific hereditary syndromes with discrete gene mutations such as lymphedemadistichiasis (FOXC2), some forms of Milroy disease, and hypotrichosislymphedema-telangiectasis (SOX18).

The future holds promise that such testing, combined with careful phenotypic descriptions, will become routine to classify familial lymphangiodysplastic syndromes and other congenital/genetic-dysmorphogenic disorders characterized by lymphedema, lymphangiectasia, and lymphangiomatosis. In addition, there are many other clinical syndromes with lymphedema as a component, and these may have genes identified in the future. The emerging era of molecular lymphology will result in improved understanding, evaluation and treatment in clinical lymphology; dramatic progress has been made towards effective targeted molecular therapies for lymphedema. Vascular endothelial growth factors C (VEGF-C) and their receptors (VEGFR-3) are known to be the primary players, but these molecules work in sync with other factors. Currently, no specific molecular treatment options are available for clinical use; however, promising results from animal trials suggest a role for VEGF-C gene therapy in treatment of lymphedema. Other results indicate that other factors such as COX-2, MMP-9, and interstitial flow dynamics may also be important in future management of lymphedema. Combination therapies such as stem cell implantation, skin grafting, and lymph node transfer in conjunction with VEGF-C therapy may further expand the effectiveness of future therapies as well. Design of a drug to treat lymphedema will require an effective animal model that accurately mimics lymphedema in humans, and further evaluation of the metastatic risk of inducing lymphangiogenesis in cancer patients is also needed. Due to the proliferative efforts of researchers over the last decade, effective treatments for lymphedema in humans may soon be a reality. However, while the addition of growth (or inhibitory) factors is attractive, the availability of these treatments in the future is uncertain at this time and should be conducted in the context of co-morbid conditions (presence of cancer, cancer treatments, drug regimens).

The second group of primary lymphedema is lymphedema praecox (Meige disease) that represents 80 per cent of primary lymphedema and occurs (estimated incidence 1.15 in 100,000 people younger than 20) after birth but before the age of 35. The age of onset is generally in adolescence (Wheeler, et al 1981). There is, unfortunately, no cure but, occasionally, patients will improve with time. BOTOX injections may help with the blepharospasm and can be used to suppress mouth movements but it is no cure. Some patients are benefited by anticholinergics such as Artane (trihexphenidyl) or Cogentin (benztropine) and few are benefited by muscle relaxants such as Lioresal (baclofen). Anti-convulsants such as Tegretol (carbamazepine) have also been employed with sporadic benefit. The only causative genes so far identified for the non-congenital primary lymphoedemas are the transcription factor FOXC2, where mutations are known to produce lymphoedema with distichiasis, and SOX18 in the very rare condition hypotrichosis-lymphoedema-telangiectasia. A recent study has examined the FOXC2 gene by sequence analysis in 23 affected individuals with Meige disease (Rezaie et al, 2008). A novel truncating mutation (c.563-584del) was identified in one family and found to segregate with the disease in eight affected relatives over three generations. Although the affected patient, initially selected for mutation screening from this family, had lymphoedema without distichiasis, all but one of his affected relatives who carried the FOXC2 mutation did have accessory eyelashes originating from their meibomian glands. This is further confirmation that of the primary lymphoedemas, only lymphoedema with distichiasis is caused by FOXC2 mutations.

The third group of primary lymphedema is lymphedema tarda. It occurs in individuals older than 35 years (Kinmonth et al, 1957). Out of all patients with primary lymphedema, 10 per cent have lymphedema tarda. The cause of lymphedema tarda is a break in the FOXC2 gene. Decongestive therapy is the most widely accepted form of treatment. Today there is no cure for lymphedema tarda, but the condition can be managed by early diagnosis and treatment.

Even in this group, the emerging era of molecular lymphology will result in improved understanding, evaluation and treatment in clinical lymphology.

Secondary lymphedema develops as a consequence of disruption or obstruction of the lymphatic pathways by surgery or other disease processes. Secondary lymphedema is much more common than the primary form. Its global incidence can be ascribed, predominantly, to filariasis, which accounts for over 90 million afflicted individuals (Laharya et al, 2011). Nevertheless, there is a growing number of lymphedema cases that are arising as a consequence of neoplastic disease, both through direct lymphatic invasion and, iatrogenically, through treatment of the neoplasm. It has been reported to occur within days and up to 30 years after treatment for breast cancer (Shaw et al, 2007). Cancer rates could further increase by 50 per cent to 15 million new cases in the year 2020 and we can assume that incidences of lymphedema will increase in the future. The most frequent causes are breast cancer in lymphedema of the arm, and prostate cancer in disease of the leg (Smith et al, 1963). In rare cases, lymphedema can lead to a form of cancer called lymphangiosarcoma, although the mechanism of carcinogenesis is not understood. Lymphedema-associated lymphangiosarcoma is called Stewart-Treves syndrome. Lymphangiosarcoma most frequently occurs in cases of long-standing lymphedema. The incidence of angiosarcoma is estimated to be 0.45 per cent in patients living five years after radical mastectomy (Chopra 2007). Lymphedema is also associated with a low-grade form of cancer called retiform hemangioendothelioma (a low-grade angiosarcoma).

Moreover, another rare case of lymphedema is the Yellow nail syndrome, defined (Samman and White 1964) as a combination of slow growing, discoloured nails. In this book Fredrik Berglund deal with this rare syndrome referring to several papers which mention the exposure to titanium implants and titanium dioxe preceding the development of yellow nails and also return to normal conditions after withdrawal of the drugs. The author suggests that nail changes and defective lymph drainage are related, and considers that "nail changes are believed to be the result of defective lymph drainage". Since titanium is always present in the nails of these patients, it is more tempting to consider the nail changes as a toxic reaction to titanium. Since lymphedema is disfiguring, causes difficulties in daily living and can lead to lifestyle becoming severely limited, it may also result in psychological distress.

Gabriella Wernicke, as a board certified radiation oncologist, presents a careful review about the lymphedema in post-operative breast cancer. In 2008, the American Cancer Society published the results of this study entitled "Preoperative Assessment Enables the Early Diagnosis and Successful Treatment of Lymphedema". The study revealed that early diagnosis of lymphedema in breast cancer patients (called stage 0 in the article) associated with an early intervention, a compression sleeve and gauntlet for one month, led to a return to pre-operative baseline status. In a five year follow-up, patients remained at their preoperative baseline, suggesting that preclinical detection of lymphedema can halt if not reverse its progression (Stout Gergich et al, 2008).

The chapter: "Preparing for and Coping with Breast Cancer-related Lymphedema", is aimed at addressing real and present concerns for both patients and their family members regarding breast cancer-related lymphedema. Research interests include roles of patients in familial and social relationships within the specific context of their own family members' or friends' illness experiences with emphasis on lymphedema and lymphedema-related symptoms.

The group of Fondazione IRCCS "Istituto dei tumori" of Milan presents an innovative theory on a new model of lymphedema: pelvic lymphedema

This lymphedema might be a consequence of mechanical pelvic injury or of the altered lymphatic system caused by such injury. The extra-peritoneal pelvic area is sited between the peritoneum, covering the pelvic organs, and the pelvic diaphragm. In the pelvic cavity the peritoneum is separated from the walls which delimit the cavity by the surrounding and supporting fatty extra-peritoneal tissue. Pelvic lymphadenectomy may lead to damaged lymphatic vessels with subsequent pelvic malfunction within a few weeks post-surgery, if undiagnosed and untreated, and can progress to a chronic pelvic dysfunction (Vannelli et al, 2009).

In conclusion I recommend remembering that "but even if the old masters have discovered everything, one thing will be always new - the application and the scientific study and classification of the discoveries made by others." (Gummere, 1917-28). Lymphangiogenesis is a complex process that involves the interplay of many molecules with redundant mechanisms and, though a solid body of evidence exists, significant research is ultimately still needed. Moreover, to date, lymphedema is frequently undiagnosed even in teaching centres (Schuchhardt C, 1997), and it seems likely that many surgical interventions have not been adequately studied with respect to lymphatic damage and their consequences. Is the future of lymphedema near? Clarke's Second Law is: "The only way of discovering the limits of the possible is to venture a little way past them into the impossible" (Clarke, 1962). Lymphedema issues this challenge.

5. References

Ambrose, C. (2006). Immunology's first priority dispute—An account of the 17th-century Rudbeck–Bartholin feud. *Cellular Immunology*, Vol.242, N.1, (July 2006), pp. 1-8, ISSN 1672-7681

Arvy, L. & Rivet, R. (1976). Marie Philibert Constant Sappey (1810-1896). The man and the lymphologist . *Bulletin De l'Association Des Anatomistes (Nancy)*, Vol.60, N.168 (March 1976), pp. 63-79, ISSN 0376-6160

Carati, C.J.; Anderson, S.N.; Gannon, B.J. & Piller, N.B. (2003). Treatment of post-mastectomy lymphedema with low-level laser therapy. *Cancer* Vol.15, N.98(6), (September 2003), pp. 1114–22, ISSN: 1097-0142

Chopra, S.; Ors, F. & Bergin, D. (2007). MRI of angiosarcoma associated with chronic lymphoedema: Stewart Treves syndrome. *British Journal of Radiology* N.80(960), (December 2007), pp. 310-3, ISSN: 1748-880X.

Clarke, AC.; (1962) Hazards of prophecy :The failure of imagination in Profiles of the Future, Harper & Row, ISBN 0-445-04061-0, New York

Dahlberg, P.J.; Borer, W.Z.; Newcomer, K.L. & Yutuc, W.R. (1983). Autosomal or X-linked recessive syndrome of congenital lymphedema, hypoparathyroidism, nephropathy, prolapsing mitral valve, and brachytelephalangy. *American Journal of Medical Genetics*. N.16(1), (September 1983), pp. 99-104, ISSN: 0148-7299

El Segundo, C.A. (2006). Low Level Laser FDA Cleared for the Treatment of Lymphedema, In: *Press Release Distribution*, Available from: http://www.prweb.com/releases/2006/12/prweb487900.htm

Fang, Y.; He, Y. & Liu, Z. (2008). Negative pressure in pharyngo-oral cavity can treat lymphedema and related disorders. *Medical Hypotheses*, Vol.70, N.4, (October 2008), pp.886-7, ISSN 0306-9877

Fanous, M.Y.; Phillips, A.J. & Windsor, J.A. (2006). Mesenteric lymph: the bridge to future management of critical illness. *Journal Of Pancreas*, Vol.9, N.8(4), (July 2007), pp. 374-99, ISSN 1590-8577

Gummere, RM. (1917-25). 3 vols. Volume I. Epistle LXIV, In: *Lucius Annaeus Seneca. Moral Epistles. Translated by Richard M. Gummere*. The Loeb Classical Library, pp. 117, Cambridge, Mass.: Harvard UP, Retrived from <http://www.stoics.com/seneca_epistles_book_1.html>

Hagelin, O. (1989). *Rare and important medical books in the library of the Swedish Society of Medicine*, Svenska Lakaresallskapet, ISBN 9781174702020, Stockholm, Swedish

Husiya, K. & Waran, Iwa. (1805). Reprinted by Teizo O (*Japan Society for History of Medicine*), Ishi Yaku Shuppan Kabushiki Gaisha ISBN: 426370441X , Tokyo, Japan

Kinmonth, J.B.; Taylor, G.W.; Tracy, G.D. & Marsh, J.D. Primary Lymphoedema. Clinical and lymphangiographic studies of a series of 107 patients in which the lower limbs were affected. British Journal of Surgery. N.45(189), (July 1957), pp.1–10, ISSN: 1365-2168

Lahariya, C.; Tomar, S.S. (2011). How endemic countries can accelerate lymphatic filariasis elimination? An analytical review to identify strategic and programmatic interventions. *Journal of Vector Borne Diseases*. N.48(1), (March 2011), pp. 1-6, ISSN:0972-9062

Luyendijk-Elshout, A.M. (1964). *Introduction in: Dilucidatio valvularam in vasis lymphaticis et lacteis*. In Dutch Classics on History of Science, XI, Ed. B. De Graaf, ISBN: 9060044290, Nieuwkoop, Netherland

National Lymphedema Network Medical Advisor Committee. (2011). In: *Position statement of the national lymphedema network*, 20 November 2010, Available from: http://www.lymphnet.org/pdfDocs/nlntreatment.pdf

Norman, J. (1978). *Medicine and the life sciences*. In Catalogue No.4, Jeremy Norman & Co, Inc, ISBN : 0825617103 9780825617102, San Francisco, United State of America

Pecquet, J. (1651). *Experimenta nova anatomica, quibus incognitum chyli receptaculum, et ab eo per thoracem in ramos usque subclavis vasa lactea deteguntur*, Apud Sebastianum Cramoisy et Gabrielem Cramoisy, Paris, France

Purushotham, AD.; Bennett Britton, TM.; Klevesath, MB.; Chou, P.; Agbaje, OF. & Duffy, SW. (2007). Lymph node status and breast cancer-related lymphedema. *Annal of Surgery*, Vol.246, N.1, (July 2007), pp. 42-5, ISSN 1528-1140

Regis, O. & Kaoru M. (1997). Paolo Mascagni, Ernest Alexandra Lauth and Marie Philibert Constant Sappey on the Dissection and Injection of the Lymphatics. *Journal of the International Society for Plastination,* Vol.12, N.2 (February 1997), pp. 4-7, ISSN 1090-2171

Rezaie, T.; Ghoroghchian ,R.; Bell, R.; Brice, G.; Hasan, A.; Burnand, K.; Vernon, S.; Mansour, S.; Mortimer, P.; Jeffery, S.; Child, A. & Sarfarazi, M. (2008), Primary non-syndromic lymphoedema (Meige disease) is not caused by mutations in FOXC2. *European Journal of Human Genetics.* N.16(3), (March 2008), pp. 300-4, ISSN: 1018-4813

Rouviere, P.H. (1932). *Anatomie des lymphatiques de l'homme,* Masson et Cie, ISBN 0-8016-3556-X, Paris, France

Ruysch, F. (1665). *Dilucidatio valvularum in vasis lymphaticis et lacteis,* ex officina Harmani Gael, Hagae Comitis, Netherland

Schuchhardt, C. (1997). Lymphedema. An easy diagnosis - but frequently missed. *Fortschritte der Medizin,* Vol. 20, N.115, (August 1997), pp. 24, 27-31, ISSN 0946-5634

Shaw, C.; Mortimer, P.; Judd, P.A.; (2007). Randomized controlled trial comparing a low-fat diet with a weight-reduction diet in breast cancer-related lymphedema. *Cancer* Vol.15, N.109 (10), (May 2007), pp. 1949-56, ISSN: 1097-0142

Smith, R.D.; Spittell, J.A. & Schirger, A. (1963). Secondary lymphedema of the leg: its characteristics and diagnostic implications. *Journal of the American Medical Association.* N.185, (July 1963), pp. 116–18 ISSN: 1538-3598

Stout Gergich, N.L.; Pfalzer, L.A.; McGarvey, C.; Springer, B.; Gerber, L.H. & Soballe, P. (2008). Pre-operative assessment enables the early diagnosis and successful treatment of lymphedema. *Cancer,* Vol.15, N.112(12), (June 2008), pp. 2809-19 ISSN: 1097-0142

Szuba, A.; Achalu, R. & Rockson, S.G. (2002). Decongestive lymphatic therapy for patients with breast carcinoma-associated lymphedema. A randomized, prospective study of a role for adjunctive intermittent pneumatic compression. *Cancer,* Vol.1, N.95(11), (December 2002), pp.2260-7, ISSN: 1097-0142

Vannelli, A.; Battaglia, L.; Poiasina, E. & Leo E. Pelvic lymphedema: Truth or fiction? *Medical Hypotheses,* Vol.72, N.3, (March 2009), pp. 267-70, ISSN 0306-9877

Warren, AG.; Brorson, H.; Borud, LJ. & Slavin, SA. (2007). Lymphedema - a comprehensive review. *Annals of Plastic Surgery,* Vol.59, N.4, (October 2007), pp. 464-72, ISSN 1536-3708

Wheeler, E.S.; Chan, V.; Wassman, R.; Rimoin, D.L. & Lesavoy, M.A. (1981). Familial lymphedema praecox: Meige's disease. *Plastic and Reconstructive Surgery.* N.67(3), (March 1981), pp. 362-4, ISSN: 1529-4242

1

Strategies in Modulating Lymphedema

Jin-Hong Chang*, Joshua H. Hou, Sandeep Jain and Dimitri T. Azar*
Department of Ophthalmology and Visual Sciences, University of Illinois Chicago
United States of America

1. Introduction

Lymphedema is the accumulation of interstitial fluid within tissues due to the impairment of lymphatic function. Dysfunction can result from direct obstruction of lymphatic vessels, absence of lymphatic vessels, or inadequate lymphatic function. From congenital forms of lymphedema, such as Milroy disease, to acquired forms of lymphedema, such as filiarisis lymphedema or post-surgical lymphedema, lymphatic dysfunction contributes significantly to the world's human disease burden.

Due to the inherent difficulties in visualizing lymphatic channels, research in the pathogenesis and treatment of lymphedema has lagged behind similar investigations in vascular pathology. Over the past two decades, aggressive research efforts have vastly improved our understanding of the lymphatic system, but significant advances in medical therapies for lymphedema and lymphatic regeneration are still lacking. To date, the majority of treatment strategies for lymphedema (compression stockings, massage, and exercise) do not address the underlying molecular pathophysiology (Nakamura & Rockson, 2008).

Several nonspecific pharmacological agents, such as selenium and benzo-pyrones, have been studied with limited success. A review of ten different trials of pharmacological therapies for lymphedema by Kligman *et al.* concluded that insufficient evidence exists to support the use of these nonspecific medical therapies at the moment (Kligman et al., 2004).

With improvements in our understanding of the molecular mechanisms of lymphedema and lymphangiogenesis, however, an increasing number of potential pharmacological targets for specific therapies are being identified. Due to ongoing efforts by numerous researchers in the study of therapeutic lymphatic regeneration, significant progress is being made towards targeted pharmacological therapies for lymphedema. Specific molecules that have shown the most promise as therapeutic targets include the vascular endothelial growth factors (VEGFs) and their receptors (VEGFRs), cyclooxygenase 2 (COX-2) selective inhibitors, tumor necrosis factor (TNF)-α, and transforming growth factor (TGF)-β.

---

*Corresponding author

2. Nonspecific treatments

To date, studies have been unable to confirm the effectiveness of nonspecific treatment strategies such as selenium and benzo-pyrones on lymphedema, despite their common use in clinical practice. Selenium is a drug that is used to prevent or minimize the adverse effects of radiotherapy, chemotherapy, or surgery in oncology patients; however, after rigorous testing of this therapy, Dennert and Horneber concluded that inadequate evidence exists to advocate for or against the use of selenium for lymphedema (Dennert & Horneber, 2006). Similarly, benzo-pyrones have been considered a plausible treatment strategy for lymphedema, as these molecules reduce vascular permeability and thereby, reduce subcutaneous fluid. Furthermore, benzo-pyrones also increase macrophage activity and encourage protein degradation, which, in turn, reduces the formation of fibrotic tissue in the lymphedematous limb. A recent review of 15 trials of benzo-pyrones in the treatment lymphedema, however, failed to uncover any conclusions due to the poor quality of the analyzed trials (Badger et al., 2004). The limited and questionable efficacy of current nonspecific treatments has led many researchers toward using molecular strategies for the development of newer targeted pharmacological therapies. Specific attention has been paid to factors responsible for lymphangiogenesis, such as VEGF-C. By stimulating lymphangiogenesis and regeneration of lost or damaged lymphatics, VEGF-C offers significant promise as a treatment for all-cause lymphedema.

3. Targeted therapies

Currently, a number of molecular strategies for the treatment of lymphedema are being studied in animal models. Promising results have been obtained in the treatment of mouse models of lymphedema via methods of promoting lymphangiogenesis; however, significant work is still required before clinical application of these therapies becomes a reality.

3.1 Treatment with VEGF-C

In particular, VEGF-C has been found to be a potent regulator of lymphangiogenesis through its actions on two receptor tyrosine kinases, VEGFR-2 and VEGFR-3 (Haiko et al., 2008; Tammela et al., 2011). Multiple studies have evaluated the efficacy of VEGF-C gene therapy and plasmid transfection and revealed surprising success in a variety of animal lymphedema models.

The first study to document improvement in the clinical and pathologic features of lymphedema by therapeutic enhancement of lymphatic drainage with human VEGF-C gene therapy was performed in 2003 by Yoon *et al*. In two animal models, a rabbit ear model and a mouse tail model, these authors treated lymphedema with naked plasmid DNA that encoded human VEGF-C (phVEGF-C) injected subcutaneously. Following treatment, improvements in both lymphedema and lymphatic function were noted (Yoon et al., 2003).

Cheung *et al*. similarly found improvement in surgically-induced lymphedema in a mouse tail model using recombinant human VEGF-C. Mice were treated with cautery ablation of the large collecting lymphatics of the tail after identification of the vessels with injected methylene blue. A lymphedematous state was then documented by evidence of dilated cutaneous lymphatics, acute inflammation and hypercellularity, and impairment of immune trafficking via *in vivo* bioluminescent imaging. Three days post-surgery, the animals were then treated with parenteral recombinant human VEGF-C generated from engineered DNA encoding the human VEGF homology domain (amino acid residues Thr103-Arg227) fused to a human CD33 signal peptide at the N-terminus and a 10x-histidine tag at the C-terminus. Upon examination, treated animals were found to have reversal of the lymphedematous state to the normal state with resolution of edema, hypercellularity, inflammatory changes, and microlymphatic dilation. Both lymphatic vessel number and cross-sectional area were reduced following exogenous administration of the recombinant VEGF-C (Cheung et al., 2006).

In another mouse model of chronic obstructive lymphedema, treatment with VEGF-C also improved lymphedema in the studied animals. The authors injected a pcDNA3.1-VEGF-C plasmid into the tail of these mice. Subsequent overexpression of VEGF-C enhanced lymphangiogenesis *in vivo* and improved lymphedema (Hu et al., 2008).

Using a rat hind limb model of lymphedema, Liu *et al.* also observed significant improvement in lymphedema following focal transfection with VEGF-C DNA. Rats were treated with a plasmid DNA encoding human VEGF-C (pcDNA3.1-VEGF-C) and monitored for resolution of their surgically-induced lymphedema in comparison to controls. Lymphedema was quantitatively reduced at 2 and 4 weeks in the therapy group as documented by magnetic resonance imaging (MRI), B-scan ultrasound, and water displacement volumetry measurements. Furthermore, numerous newly formed lymphatic vessels were observed in treated mice on both histological and immunofluorescence analysis (Liu et al., 2008).

Finally, Tammela *et al.* found a significant role for adenovirally-delivered VEGF-C in improving outcomes of lymph node dissection and transplantation in mice. In their study, lymph node dissection and transplantation in combination with adenovirally-delivered VEGF-C induced the formation of functional collecting lymphatic vessels and the reconstitution of a functional immunological barrier (Tammela et al., 2007).

3.2 Caveats to VEGF-C Therapies

Despite the growing body of evidence in support of the efficacy of VEGF-C gene therapy, the exact mechanism by which VEGF-C-induced lymphangiogenesis facilitates resolution of lymphedema remains controversial. In an effort to elucidate the mechanisms by which VEGF-C induces lymphatic microvascular remodeling, Jin *et al.* examined the effects of anti-VEGFR-3 neutralizing antibodies in a mouse tail model of post-surgical lymphedema. This study demonstrated that VEGFR-3 plays a central mechanistic role in lymphedema remodeling. In the presence of the neutralizing antibody, lymphatic remodeling was greatly attenuated due to blockage of VEGF-C-induced signaling (Jin da et al., 2009).

In contrast, Uzarski *et al.* failed to observe inhibition of edema resolution across surgically-induced wounds in a mouse tail lymphedema model upon blockage of VEGFR-3. In their study, two mouse models were compared. In the first mouse model, scar-free lymphatic obstruction was simulated with dissection and removal of the superficial lymphatics from a mouse tail. Distal lymphedema was noted, and resolution was stimulated by VEGF-C. Edema resolution was not, however, inhibited by VEGFR-3 neutralizing antibodies, although lymphangiogenesis was reduced. In the second mouse model, scar-containing lymphatic obstruction was simulated with dissection and removal of the superficial lymphatics with cautery. Subsequent treatment with either VEGF-C or VEGFR-3 neutralizing antibodies resulted in no improvement in lymphedema. The authors concluded that interstitial flow dynamics and lymphedema may actually be more dependent on the extracellular matrix that reforms at the site of the injury than on lymphangiogenesis and that this effect may be impeded by the formation of scar tissue (Uzarski et al., 2008).

Following the finding that resolution of lymphedema may be more dependent on interstitial flow than on VEGFR-3 or VEGF-C, Ongstad *et al.* set out to clarify the role of VEGFR signaling during edema resolution and to probe the mechanism by which VEGF-C hastens resolution of edema. In their study, inhibition of VEGFR-3 or VEGFR-2 alone in mouse models did not significantly change the evolution of lymphedema relative to controls; however, inhibition of both VEGFR-2 and VEGFR-3 led to reduced tissue repair and reduced resolution of tail swelling at 40 and 50 days post surgery. Thus, tissue repair was crucial to the resolution of edema as this process provides a matrix bridge for fluid drainage. These authors then hypothesized that edema resolution in the mouse may be VEGFR signaling dependent, but lymphangiogenesis independent (Ongstad et al.).

Careful analysis by Jin *et al.* identified 120 mouse genes, many of which share homology with human genes, that are upregulated in the presence of lymphedema and normalized following therapeutic VEGF-C administration. Many of these genes were found to be involved in processes unrelated to lymphangiogenesis, suggesting an underlying, but incompletely understood, complexity to VEGF-C-induced lymphedema resolution. It is likely that numerous processes, including inflammation, immune response, wound healing, angiogenesis, oxidative stress response, and adipogenesis, play important roles in the pathogenesis and therapeutic resolution of the disease (Jin da et al., 2009). Additional research in this area is certainly warranted.

3.3 VEGF-C and stem cell combined therapies

Several recent studies further complicated our understanding of the role of VEGF-C and the optimal application of VEGF-C therapy in the treatment of lymphedema. In two papers, augmentation strategies using synthetic extracellular matrix material, such as gelatin and/or stem cells, co-administered with VEGF-C resulted in greater resolution of lymphedema compared to VEGF-C therapy alone. This further highlights the complexity of lymphedema and VEGF-C therapy.

Gelatin is a natural and abundant polymer used for tissue engineering. Gelatin-based hydrogels are biodegradable, non-immunogenic, and non-toxic and are able to mimic the properties of the extracellular matrix. This polymer can be used to distribute growth factors in a localized, sustained, controlled manner to obtain an effective dose response. Due to these properties and the success of VEGF-C treatment in lymphedema mouse models, Hwang *et al.* created a mouse hind limb model of lymphedema and applied a gelatin hydrogel system to the site of injury to obtain a controlled release of VEGF-C in combination with injection of human adipose-derived stem cells (hADSCs). Decreased dermal edema depth and increased lymphatic vessel density were observed at all time periods in the mice treated with both hydrogel and hADSCs as compared to mice treated with either hydrogel or hADSCs alone (Hwang et al.)

Similarly, Zhou *et al.* treated rabbits with hind limb lymphedema using bone marrow stromal cells and/or VEGF-C. The rabbits that were treated with both stem cells and the growth factor exhibited a significant decrease in volume of edema in the limb as compared to rabbits treated with only one of the two agents. Vessel numbers increased in the dual treatment group, and VEGF-C expression was also higher in the dual therapy-treated animals. The authors concluded that the treatments enhanced the therapeutic effect of each other (Hu et al.). Therefore, stem cells may play a role in matrix remodeling and lymphangiogenesis, particularly in the setting of upregulated VEGF-C expression; however, further research is needed before concrete conclusions can be made.

3.4 Alternative therapies

As our understanding of lymphatics has improved, additional therapies with effects on lymphangiogenesis have also been identified. One such therapy is extracorporeal shock wave therapy (ECT). ECT is used for the treatment of plantar fasciitis and tennis elbow. Repeated shock waves are localized to an area to produce neo-vascularization. This treatment effectively induces therapeutic angiogenesis and improves myocardial ischemia in pigs and humans as well as hind limb ischemia in rabbits via a mechanism involving upregulation of VEGF. Serizawa *et al.* created a rat tail model of lymphedema and subsequently subjected the animals to serial ECT therapy. Enhanced drainage of lymphatic fluid as well as upregulation of VEGF-C expression were found in the treatment group compared to the controls (Serizawa et al.).

Similarly, skin graft repairs to injuries in a mouse tail model have also been shown to stimulate lymphatic regeneration. In a recent study by Yan *et al.*, ingrowth of lymphatic vessels and spontaneous re-connection of existing lymphatics associated with VEGF-C up-regulation was observed following skin grafting (Avraham et al.). In the future, a combination of such therapeutic strategies may be required for optimal management of lymphedema.

3.5 Additional molecular targets

Clearly, VEGF-C plays an important role in the lymphatic system; however, it is also becoming increasingly clear that additional factors are involved in lymphedema. One such factor, hepatocyte growth factor (HGF), has been found to promote lymphatic vessel formation in mice. Furthermore, both HGF and its high affinity HGF receptor (MET) have recently been found to be expressed in lymphatic endothelial cells but not in blood endothelial cells. Finegold *et al.* examined these genes in women with secondary lymphedema following treatment for breast cancer and found that patients with both primary and secondary lymphedema had mutations in HGF/MET, suggesting that mutations in HGF/MET may be a significant risk factor for lymphedema. Thus, HGF may also become a potent therapeutic target for the treatment of lymphedema (Finegold et al., 2008).

Another potential new target for lymphedema therapy is matrix metalloproteinase (MMP)-9. Sustained swelling induced by lymphatic ligation leads to lymphatic hyperplasia and VEGF-C upregulation; however, mice lacking MMP-9 have a larger increase in tail volume with secondary lymphedema as compared to wild-type mice (Rutkowski et al., 2006).

G-protein-coupled receptors are expressed during lymphatic development and function, and thus, these molecules are also potential targets for pharmacological treatment. Genetically engineered mouse models deficient in specific G-protein-coupled receptors have been used to identify several specific G-proteins, such as the adrenomedullin receptor, that are important for lymphatic vascular development and function (Dunworth & Caron, 2009).

Radiation therapy, infections, or extensive surgical resection promote scarring and fibrosis and are, thus, also risk factors for lymphedema. Based on this finding, Avraham *et al.* examined the specific impact of fibrosis, defined as the excessive deposition of extracellular matrix products, on the abnormal regeneration of lymphatic vessels. Inhibition of fibrosis via treatment of the mouse tails with collagen type 1 gel and a moist dressing accelerated lymphatic regeneration and reduced post-surgical acute lymphedema in this animal model. Lymphatic endothelial cell proliferation was also enhanced and lymphatic function was improved. These results were independent of VEGF-C expression (Avraham et al., 2009).

After discovering that fibrosis impairs lymphatic regeneration and function (Avraham et al., 2009), Avraham *et al.* then searched for factors that modulate fibrosis in lymphedemous tissue. Transforming growth factor (TGF)-β is a well-known regulator of extracellular matrix synthesis. Inhibition of TGF-β causes both decreased fibrosis in virtually every organ system and increased lymphatic endothelial cell proliferation, migration, and tubule formation. To study the role of TGF-β, the investigators compared biopsies from lymphedemous limbs of patients to biopsies of the normal contralateral limb. The limbs with lymphedema exhibited a 3-fold increase in the number of TGF-β1-positive cells as compared to the normal limbs. Similarly, a mouse tail model of lymphedema was studied to determine the effect of anti-TGF-β1 treatment on lymphedema. Application of a TGF-β1 antibody (TGFmab) induced a 50-60% decrease in tail volume (a surrogate measurement for lymphedema) in treated mice compared to control mice. The treatment was well tolerated with no evidence of toxicity or wound healing complications. In the future, blockage of TGF-β may lead to further therapeutic options for augmentation of lymphatic regeneration. (Avraham et al., 2010).

Lymphedema has also been found to arise from destructive tissue injury independent of lymph stasis. Based on this observation, inflammatory mediators such as tumor necrosis factor (TNF)-α and cyclooxygenase (COX) have also come under recent scrutiny. TNF-α is prominently expressed in lymphedematous tissue in mouse models and is a known inducer of VEGF-C expression. In a mouse tail model of lymphedema, Nakamura *et al.* examined the anti-inflammatory and possible lymphangiogenic potential of a non-steroidal anti-inflammatory drug (NSAID) and a modified soluble form of a TNF-α receptor R1 (sTNF-R1) on TNF-α expression. Subcutaneous injections of the NSAID ketoprofen, which reduces inflammation by inhibiting COX but increases TNF-α levels, resulted in marked improvement in inflammation, normalization of histological changes, and disappearance of dilated microlymphatics with associated up-regulation TNF-α expression. Treatment with the NSAID also led to upregulation of VEGF-C, VEGFR-3, and Prox1, all factors associated with lymphangiogenesis. Treatment of mice with sTNF-R1, which directly inactivates TNF-α and downregulates its expression, did not result in improvement in lymphedema, and epidermal thickness actually increased in treated mice compared to untreated mice. In these treated mice, both VEGF-C and VEGFR-3 expression decreased as well. Though more evidence is needed, TNF-α activity and its downstream effects on VEGF-C may actually be a protective response to injury-induced lymphedema (Nakamura et al., 2009).

In contrast, another study revealed that increased COX-2 expression was associated with recurrence of lymph flow in wound granulation tissues and with increased formation of lymphatic vessel endothelial hyaluronan receptor 1 (LYVE-1)-positive lymphatic-like structures. The authors suggest that these results differed from those of Nakamura *et al.* as a result of the important selectivity of the COX inhibitors (Kashiwagi et al., 2011). Thus, the role of inflammatory mediators, such as TNF-α and COX-2, in the treatment of lymphedema remains both complex and controversial.

4. Larger animal models

Most animal models of lymphedema are mouse models due to the practicalities of establishing new treatment methods; however, utilizing mice carries significant limitations. The microlymphatics in the superficial dermis of mouse tails and the complex macrostructure of human lymphatics, which includes both larger collecting vessels and lymph nodes, have notable differences that preclude direct correlation. Extrapolation of the therapeutic successes achieved in mice to humans, therefore, is dangerous without further experimentation in larger animals.

To that end, Lahteenvuo *et al.* recently investigated the benefits of adenoviral vector-assisted VEGF-C gene therapy in the treatment of lymphedema in pigs. Lymphedema was induced in pigs by excising a 3 cm piece of the inguinal lymphatic vessels that drain distally and proximally from the inguinal lymph node. The pedicular lymph node was then reattached to the remaining tissue 4 cm laterally from its original position, thereby mimicking lymph node transfer in human patients. Adenoviral vectors encoding full-length VEGF-C were then injected into the lymph node. Following injection, expression of VEGF-C was significantly increased. Furthermore, survival and functionality of the transferred lymph nodes was markedly improved in the injected animals as compared to the controls. Lymph node transfer has been used in humans with limited success (22-31%), but in this model, the presence of VEGF-C resulted in better lymphatic vessel function, collecting vessel formation, and lymph node histology compared to controls (Lahteenvuo et al., 2011).

Similar studies have also been performed on other large animals such as sheep. Using such a model, Baker *et al.* tested the effect of lymphangiogenic growth factors delivered via slow-release diffusion on the resolution of lymphedema after lymph node extraction. A single popliteal lymph node was extracted from the sheep to induce distal limb lymphedema. Hydrogel HAMC (a blend of hyaluronan and methylcellulose that facilitates slow protein diffusion) infused with VEGF-C and angiopoietin-2 was then injected into the excision site. The animals that received treatment displayed significantly reduced edema compared with the untreated animals (Baker et al.).

Though no formal testing of targeted therapies for lymphedema has been performed in humans to date, a few isolated case reports have been published. Sorafenib, a synthetic compound produced to block the enzyme RAF-kinase, was found to cause a dramatic reduction in chronic lymphedema in one human case study. As part of a clinical study, the patient took 400 mg of sorafenib twice daily, and the lymphedema was dramatically reduced within a few days of starting treatment. The effect was directly proportional to the dose and was not sustained when the drug was discontinued due to other side effects. The authors hypothesized that the reduction of lymphedema was due to VEGFR-2 blockade, which reduced vascular permeability but did not affect the VEGFR-3 pathway involved in the proliferation of lymphatic endothelial cells (Moncrieff et al., 2008).

5. Limitations

Though research into targeted therapies for lymphedema is progressing rapidly, significant work is still required. As stated above, there are a number of limitations with the animal models that are currently available. First, the models are based on acute lymphatic damage and not on chronic lymphedema. Lymphedema in humans is slowly progressive and does not recover naturally, whereas the models that are studied progress quickly and often regress naturally. Rats, for example, heal very quickly, and tail lymphedema heals itself. In fact, one of the problems in studying lymphedema treatment strategies is the difficulty in developing a method to sustain lymphedema long enough to study the outcomes of the therapies (Yoon et al., 2003). In addition, the hydrostatic conditions of humans differ from those of small animals, such as mice, rats, and rabbits, that are usually used to study lymphedema. The absolute lymphatic area damaged in humans is greater than in these small animals, and the regenerating lymphatic vessels must span a longer distance. Models using pigs, which are closer in size to humans, will likely be useful in addressing some of these issues. Another major concern is that VEGF-C and VEGFR-3 are known to promote metastasis. Since a large portion of lymphedema patients are breast cancer survivors, an understanding of the metastatic risks associated with VEGF-C treatment of lymphedema is of paramount importance. However, these potentially damaging side effects of VEGF-C treatment are difficult to study in animal models.

6. Conclusion

Lymphangiogenesis is a complex process that involves the interplay of many molecules with redundant mechanisms. VEGF-C and VEGFR-3 are known to be the primary players, but these molecules work in sync with other factors. Currently, no specific molecular treatment options are available for clinical use; however, promising results from animal trials suggest a role for VEGF-C gene therapy in treatment of lymphedema. Other results indicate that other factors such as COX-2, MMP-9, and interstitial flow dynamics may also be important in future management of lymphedema. Combination therapies such as stem cell implantation, skin grafting, and lymph node transfer in conjunction with VEGF-C therapy may further expand the effectiveness of future therapies as well. Design of a drug to treat lymphedema will require an effective animal model that accurately mimics lymphedema in humans. And further evaluation of the metastatic risk of inducing lymphangiogenesis in cancer patients is also needed. However, dramatic progress has been made towards effective targeted molecular therapies for lymphedema. Due to the proliferative efforts of researchers over the last decade, effective treatments for lymphedema in humans may soon be a reality. However, though a solid body of evidence now exists in support of targeted therapies for lymphedema, significant research is ultimately still needed.

7. References

Avraham, T., Clavin, N.W., Daluvoy, S.V., Fernandez, J., Soares, M.A., Cordeiro, A.P., & Mehrara, B.J. (2009). Fibrosis is a key inhibitor of lymphatic regeneration. *Plastic and Reconstructive Surgery*, Vol.124, No.2, pp. 438-450.

Avraham, T., Daluvoy, S., Zampell, J., Yan, A., Haviv, Y.S., Rockson, S.G., & Mehrara, B.J. (2010). Blockade of transforming growth factor-beta1 accelerates lymphatic regeneration during wound repair. *The American Journal of Pathology*, Vol.177, No.6, pp. 3202-3214.

Badger, C., Preston, N., Seers, K., & Mortimer, P. (2004). Benzo-pyrones for reducing and controlling lymphoedema of the limbs. *Cochrane Database Syst Rev*, Vol.2, CD003140.

Baker, A., Kim, H., Semple, J.L., Dumont, D., Shoichet, M., Tobbia, D., & Johnston, M. (2010). Experimental assessment of pro-lymphangiogenic growth factors in the treatment of post-surgical lymphedema following lymphadenectomy. *Breast Cancer Research*, Vol.12, No.5, R70.

Cheung, L., Han, J., Beilhack, A., Joshi, S., Wilburn, P., Dua, A., An, A., & Rockson, S.G. (2006). An experimental model for the study of lymphedema and its response to therapeutic lymphangiogenesis. *BioDrugs*, Vol.20, No.6, pp. 363-370.

Dennert, G., & Horneber, M. (2006). Selenium for alleviating the side effects of chemotherapy, radiotherapy and surgery in cancer patients. *Cochrane Database Syst Rev*, Vol.3, CD005037.

Dunworth, W.P., & Caron, K.M. (2009). G protein-coupled receptors as potential drug targets for lymphangiogenesis and lymphatic vascular diseases. *Arteriosclerosis, Thrombosis, and Vascular Biology*, Vol.29, No.5, pp. 650-656.

Finegold, D.N., Schacht, V., Kimak, M.A., Lawrence, E.C., Foeldi, E., Karlsson, J.M., Baty, C.J., & Ferrell, R.E. (2008). HGF and MET mutations in primary and secondary lymphedema. *Lymphatic Research and Biology*, Vol.6, No.2, pp. 65-68.

Haiko, P., Makinen, T., Keskitalo, S., Taipale, J., Karkkainen, M.J., Baldwin, M.E., Stacker, S.A., Achen, M.G., & Alitalo, K. (2008). Deletion of vascular endothelial growth factor C (VEGF-C) and VEGF-D is not equivalent to VEGF receptor 3 deletion in mouse embryos. *Molecular and Cellular Biology*, Vol.28, No.15, pp. 4843-4850.

Hu, X.Q., Jiang, Z.H., & Liu, N.F. (2008). Experimental studies of VEGF-C gene for the treatment of chronic obstructive lymphedema in mouse tail model. *Chinese Journal of Plastic Surgery*, Vol.24, No.3, pp. 207-211.

Hwang, J.H., Kim, I.G., Lee, J.Y., Piao, S., Lee, D.S., Lee, T.S., & Ra, J.C. (2011). Therapeutic lymphangiogenesis using stem cell and VEGF-C hydrogel. *Biomaterials*, Vol.32, No.19, pp. 4415-4423.

Jin da, P., An, A., Liu, J., Nakamura, K., & Rockson, S.G. (2009). Therapeutic responses to exogenous VEGF-C administration in experimental lymphedema: immunohistochemical and molecular characterization. *Lymphatic Research and Biology*, Vol.7, No.1, pp. 47-57.

Kashiwagi, S., Hosono, K., Suzuki, T., Takeda, A., Uchinuma, E., & Majima, M. (2011). Role of COX-2 in lymphangiogenesis and restoration of lymphatic flow in secondary lymphedema. *Laboratory Investigation*, Vol.91, No.9, pp. 1314-1325.

Kligman, L., Wong, R.K., Johnston, M., & Laetsch, N.S. (2004). The treatment of lymphedema related to breast cancer: a systematic review and evidence summary. *Supportive Care in Cancer*, Vol.12, No.6, pp. 421-431.

Lahteenvuo, M., Honkonen, K., Tervala, T., Tammela, T., Suominen, E., Lahteenvuo, J., Kholova, I., Alitalo, K., Yla-Herttuala, S., & Saaristo, A. (2011). Growth factor therapy and autologous lymph node transfer in lymphedema. *Circulation*, Vol.123, No.6, pp. 613-620.

Liu, Y., Fang, Y., Dong, P., Gao, J., Liu, R., Tian, H., Ding, Z., Bi, Y., & Liu, Z. (2008). Effect of vascular endothelial growth factor C (VEGF-C) gene transfer in rat model of secondary lymphedema. *Vascular Pharmacology*, Vol.49, No.1, pp. 44-50.

Moncrieff, M., Shannon, K., Hong, A., Hersey, P., & Thompson, J. (2008). Dramatic reduction of chronic lymphoedema of the lower limb with sorafenib therapy. *Melanoma Research*, Vol.18, No.2, pp. 161-162.

Nakamura, K., Radhakrishnan, K., Wong, Y.M., & Rockson, S.G. (2009). Anti-inflammatory pharmacotherapy with ketoprofen ameliorates experimental lymphatic vascular insufficiency in mice. *PLoS One*, Vol.4, No.12, e8380.

Nakamura, K., & Rockson, S.G. (2008). Molecular targets for therapeutic lymphangiogenesis in lymphatic dysfunction and disease. *Lymphatic Research and Biology*, Vol.6, No.3-4, pp. 181-189.

Ongstad, E.L., Bouta, E.M., Roberts, J.E., Uzarski, J.S., Gibbs, S.E., Sabel, M.S., Cimmino, V.M., Roberts, M.A., & Goldman, J. (2010). Lymphangiogenesis-independent resolution of experimental edema. *American Journal of Physiology Heart and Circulatory Physiology*, Vol.299, No.1, pp. H46-54.

Rutkowski, J.M., Moya, M., Johannes, J., Goldman, J., & Swartz, M.A. (2006). Secondary lymphedema in the mouse tail: Lymphatic hyperplasia, VEGF-C upregulation, and the protective role of MMP-9. *Microvascular Research*, Vol.72, No.3, pp. 161-171.

Serizawa, F., Ito, K., Matsubara, M., Sato, A., Shimokawa, H., & Satomi, S. (2011). Extracorporeal shock wave therapy induces therapeutic lymphangiogenesis in a rat model of secondary lymphoedema. *European Journal of Vascular and Endovascular Surgery*, Vol.42, No.2, pp. 254-260.

Tammela, T., Saaristo, A., Holopainen, T., Lyytikka, J., Kotronen, A., Pitkonen, M., Abo-Ramadan, U., Yla-Herttuala, S., Petrova, T.V., & Alitalo, K. (2007). Therapeutic differentiation and maturation of lymphatic vessels after lymph node dissection and transplantation. *Nature Medicine*, Vol.13, No.12, pp. 1458-1466.

Tammela, T., Zarkada, G., Nurmi, H., Jakobsson, L., Heinolainen, K., Tvorogov, D., Zheng, W., Franco, C.A., Murtomaki, A., Aranda, E., *et al.* (2011). VEGFR-3 controls tip to stalk conversion at vessel fusion sites by reinforcing Notch signalling. *Nature Cell Biology*, Vol.13, No.10, pp. 1202-1213.

Uzarski, J., Drelles, M.B., Gibbs, S.E., Ongstad, E.L., Goral, J.C., McKeown, K.K., Raehl, A.M., Roberts, M.A., Pytowski, B., Smith, M.R., *et al.* (2008). The resolution of lymphedema by interstitial flow in the mouse tail skin. *American Journal of Physiology Heart and Circulatory Physiology*, Vol.294, No.3, pp. H1326-1334.

Yoon, Y.S., Murayama, T., Gravereaux, E., Tkebuchava, T., Silver, M., Curry, C., Wecker, A., Kirchmair, R., Hu, C.S., Kearney, M., *et al.* (2003). VEGF-C gene therapy augments postnatal lymphangiogenesis and ameliorates secondary lymphedema. *Journal of Clinical Investigation*, Vol.111, No.5, pp. 717-725.

2

Titanium and Yellow Nail Syndrome

Fredrik Berglund
Swedish Society of Dental Amalgam Patients, Trollhättan, Sweden

1. Introduction

Yellow nail syndrome was defined in 1964 as a combination of slow growing, discoloured nails and edema (Samman & White, 1964). The rate of growth of finger nails was less than 0.2 mm per week compared with the normal 0.5-1.2 mm per week. The nails were thickened and the cuticles were deficient. The color varied from pale yellow to slightly greenish. Onycholysis (separation of the nail from its bed) and shedding of one or more nails was mentioned. - Of the 13 patients with yellow nails 10 presented with edema, mainly in the ankles.

Subsequently, several symptoms were described and included. *Sinusitis* was reported by Wells (Wells,1966), although clearly he did not recognize it as part of the syndrome. Chronic intermittent *cough* with sputum production was reported by Zerfas (Zerfas, 1966), and in combination with *sinusitis* and *bronchitis* by Dilley et al (Dilley et al.,1968). Hiller et al. (1972) emphasized that chronic cough was a persistent finding in all their patients.

Pleural effusion in combination with lymphedema was reported in three patients by Emerson (Emerson,1966). The pleural fluid was clear, with a protein content of 4-9 mg/100 ml. The predominant cell was the lymphocyte. The effusion always re-accumulated after drainage.

Pericardial effusion in addition to pleural effusions and lymphedema was reported by Wakasa et al. (1987).

1.1 Symptom frequency in published papers

In 78 papers listed in PubMed from 1964 to 2009 there were 185 patients diagnosed with yellow nail syndrome: 18 % with yellow nails only, 42 % together with lymphedema, 21 % together with pleural effusion, and 19 % with the complete triad yellow nails-lymphedema-pleural effusion. Thus lymphedema was diagnosed totally in 61 %. Cough and sinusitis were diagnosed in 32 %.

Among several authors reporting sinusitis, some mention radiography revealing mucoid thickening of one or more sinuses (Nakielna et al, 1976, Hassard et al,1984, Camilleri, 1990, Varney et al, 1994, Cebecci et al, 2009). Varney et al. – at a Nose Clinic in London – reported that 14 out of 17 patients with yellow nail syndrome suffered severe rhinosinusitis, which predated nail changes in four, coincided with yellow nails in six, and occurred later in the remaining seven patients.

Among my patients, sinusitis and cough were the most common symptoms (Berglund & Carlmark, 2011). Several patients spontaneously mention postnasal drip and a "strange cough" as a main feature, often starting half a year after a titanium implant or start of medication with drugs containing titanium dioxide.

2. Etiology: Titanium and titanium dioxide

Since 1997 I have seen 35 patients with one or more of the symptoms or signs mentioned above. Twenty-seven patients had titanium implants, whereas eight were exposed to titanium dioxide.

Titanium in nail clippings or shed nails from the patients was analyzed by energy dispersive x-ray fluorescence (Forsell et al., 1997). It was present in the nails in concentrations varying between 1 and 170 µg/g, with a median level of 5 µg/g (Berglund & Carlmark, 2011). Shed nails had high levels (46, 41, 22 and 6 µg/g), but some nail clippings had even higher levels (170, 120 and 111 µg/g). Titanium levels do not seem to correlate with yellowness or thickness of nails. Titanium was not found in nails from healthy subjects, not even if exposed to titanium + gold (one subject) or to drugs with titanium dioxide.

In two patients titanium was analyzed in separate nail clippings of the left hand. The thumbnail had higher level (5.6 and 4.1 µg/g) than the other nails (2.8 – 3.2 and 3.1 - 4.1 µg/g, respectively). In two patients the levels in clippings from thumb and big toe were identical (1.7 µg/g) or nearly identical (1.7 versus 1.6 µg/g). In one patient the titanium level was 48 µg/g in a shed nail, but only 6.7 µg/g in fresh clippings. Nowadays I ask for clippings from the left thumbnail, except when shed nails are available.

2.1 Titanium metal

Titanium (Ti): atomic weight 47.9, atomic number 22, specific gravity 4.54. When pure, titanium is a lustrous, white metal. It is 60 % heavier than aluminum, but twice as strong. Titanium is a much harder metal than aluminum and approaches the high hardness possessed by some of the heat-treated steels, which causes some difficulties in dentistry. Its modulus of rigidity falls between that of aluminum and that of steel. The high ductility enables the use of titanium in cochlear implant electrodes. Since it is non-ferromagnetic, patients with titanium implants can be safely examined with magnetic resonance imaging.

Titanium is quite sensitive to galvanic corrosion, e.g. by other metals and fluorine. This is to be expected when comparing their reduction potentials.

2.2 Reduction potentials (Hunsburger, 1976)

Our body shows high electrical conductivity. This enables our recording of the electrocardiogram through electrodes applied to the skin. The higher resistance in the skin is abolished by perspiration (hypotonic saline). The presence of metals with different reduction potentials may give rise to galvanic phenomena within the body or across the skin. (A young man with a gold ring in one ear experienced a buzzing sensation in the ear while holding a coca-cola can for a while in his hand). Ions of different sorts can be introduced through the skin by means of electric current, so-called iontophoresis.

Reaction	Potential (Volts)
$Ti^{+2} + 2e^- \Leftrightarrow Ti$	−1.63
$TiO_2 + 4H^+ + 4e^- \Leftrightarrow Ti + 2H_2O$	−0.86
$Ag^+ + e^- \Leftrightarrow Ag$	+0.80
$Hg^{+2} + 2e^- \Leftrightarrow Hg$	+0.85
$Au^+ + e^- \Leftrightarrow Au$	+1.69
$F_2 + 2e^- \Leftrightarrow 2F^-$	+2.87

2.3 Titanium implant patients

My first patient got a titanium and a cobalt-chromium implant in her right knee. Half a year later she developed a persistent cough. Later her nails became thick and yellow, and a few nails were shed. She had gold in many of her teeth. Analysis for metals in nail clippings revealed high levels of titanium (Berglund & Carlmark, 2011). Three years later she had normal nails and no cough, but her knee implant had loosened. She got a new implant, and a year later she had her cough and yellow nails again.

The dominant cause of yellow nail syndrome in my patients was the galvanic interaction between titanium implants and gold. There were 23 females and 4 males, aged 15-86 years at onset of symptoms. Most titanium implants were in the teeth (pins or crowns) or in the jaw bones, but also in the knees and hips, or in the abdomen (clips and staples) after laparoscopic surgery. In one patient there was iontophoresis of titanium ions from titanium spectacles to gold in the teeth.

The gold electrodes were present mostly as dental inlays and crowns, but in two patients as wedding or engagement rings. Some patients reported intolerance to gold jewelry. Patch tests with gold cannot be done in titanium implant patients. In three patients amalgam, which contains silver and mercury, formed the electric circuit with titanium. I always advise patients with amalgam or titanium not to wear metal jewelry. In three patients the local application of fluoride gel caused release of titanium from titanium inlays in the teeth. In vitro, the oxidative release of titanium ions from titanium increases sharply in the presence of fluoride (Reclaru & Meyer, 1998, Strietzel et al., 1998, Schiff et al., 2002).

Most patients with titanium implants suspected metal involvement and contacted me through the Swedish Society of Dental Amalgam Patients. However, in published papers most patients were probably exposed to titanium dioxide.

2.4 Titanium dioxide: Uses and intestinal uptake

Titanium dioxide, TiO_2, is insoluble in water and acid but soluble in alkali. Because of its brightness and high refractive index it is the most widely used white pigment. Titanium dioxide is widely used in the food and drug industry as a whitening agent and is given the European food additive number E171.

After oral administration of titanium dioxide to rats, particles of titanium dioxide were present in the gut associated lymphoid tissue, but also in the liver, spleen, lungs and peritoneal tissues, but were not detected in the heart or the kidney (Jani et al., 1994).

Titanium, together with aluminum, has consistently been found in lymphoid tissue of the ileum and in mesenteric lymph glands in patients with intestinal disease and in postmortem cases with no evidence of gastrointestinal disease (Shepherd et al., 1987). After administration of gelatin capsules with 23 mg titanium dioxide (mean particle size 0.16 µm) to five male subjects, blood levels of titanium rose from 12 µg/L to 43 µg/L at 4-12 hours (Böckmann et al., 2000). The concentration/time curves were considered to be characteristic for a persorption mechanism (absorption in pores only slightly wider than the diameter of absorbed molecules).

2.5 Titanium dioxide patients

Several papers mention the exposure to drugs preceding the development of yellow nails and also return to normal conditions after withdrawal of the drugs (David-Vaudey et al., 2004). It turns out that that all the drug tablets mentioned contain titanium dioxide.

I had eight patients (4 male, 4 female, age 15-79 years at onset of symptoms) exposed to titanium dioxide, six via drug tablets, one via confectionary, and one via chewing gum. Seven had more than ten amalgam restorations in their teeth and had gastrointestinal symptoms, mostly diarrhea, that may have facilitated the absorption of titanium dioxide. A lactulose test in one patient showed increased intestinal permeability. This might explain why relatively few patients develop the syndrome. Also, some patients told me that their strange cough started only after 6 months medication. Most patients don't take their medicines (e.g. antibiotics) that long.

3. Pathogenesis

3.1 Nail changes

Samman and White (1964) suggested that nail changes and defective lymph drainage are related. Emerson (1966) even considered that "nail changes are believed to be the result of defective lymph drainage". Since titanium is always present in the nails of these patients, it is more tempting to consider the nail changes as a toxic reaction to titanium.

3.2 Lymphedema, pleural effusions and ascites; defective lymph drainage or increased vascular leakage?

Lymphangiograms, as performed in four patients with lymphedema in the legs, were interpreted as showing defective lymph drainage (Samman & White, 1964) Similar findings have been reported later (Müller et al., 1979). More recently Danielsson et al. (2006), using lymphoscintigraphy in a patient with edema, pleural effusions, hypoalbuminemia and yellow nails, found normal lymph flow and no signs of lymphatic obstruction in the lower extremities!

Emerson (1966) noted high protein content (40-90 g/L) in pleural effusion, but still considered the primary event to be defective lymph drainage, which could not handle increased lymph formation, e.g. after some infection. Protein-losing enteropathy in patients with pleural effusions, in some cases together with ascites, has also been reported (Duhra et al., 1985, Battaglia et al., 1985, Malek et al., 1996). In a patient with edema, plural effusion, hypoalbuminaemia and yellow nails, D'Allessandro et al. (2001) found a 10-fold increase in normal albumin enteric loss. Since in most cases of yellow nail syndrome the pleural fluid has a very high protein content, this reflects increased protein permeability of systemic capillaries. D'Allessandro et al claimed that "the theory of pure lymphatic block is not sufficient to explain all the clinical manifestations of yellow nail syndrome", and suggested that microangiopathy and increased microvascular filtration at different sites (pleura, liver, limbs, intestine) due to an alteration in the interstitial matrix, could play a role in addition to lymphatic abnormality.

These reports indicate that increased vascular permeability rather than lymphatic abnormality is a key factor in yellow nail syndrome.

3.3 Prenatal and neonatal manifestations

There are two reports on pregnancy in women with yellow nails and bronchitis or productive cough (Govaert et al., 1992, Slee et al., 2000). Ultrasonography demonstrated polyhydramnios and bilateral pleural effusion in the fetuses at 23 and 29 weeks of gestation, respectively. At delivery both infants were hydropic and had bilateral pleural effusions, which were treated by thoracic drainage. Following initial recovery, pleural effusion recurred 2 days after starting enteral feeding at 4 weeks of age in the first infant, but not in the second. Our interpretation is that both mothers were exposed to titanium or titanium dioxide, and that titanium was transferred across the placenta, and possibly also via maternal milk.

There are a few reports of familiar occurrence of yellow nail syndrome (Lambert et al., 2006). They might be explained by several family members consuming drugs or chewing gum containing titanium.

4. Diagnosis

Yellow discoloration of the nails is often a late sign of the syndrome and therefore not necessary for the diagnosis of yellow nail syndrome; sinusitis and cough, lymphedema and pleural effusion occurring alone or in combination may represent the same syndrome (Varney et al., 1994, Cebecci et al., 2009). The diagnosis is supported by history or evidence of exposure to titanium implants or to titanium dioxide, and can be confirmed (if necessary) by the presence of titanium in nail clippings (>1 μg/g).

5. Treatment

5.1 Titanium implants

Most often it is impossible or extremely difficult to remove titanium implants. It is usually much easier to remove the gold (in teeth, jewelry or rings). In a few patients gold removal (Berglund & Carlmark, 2011) has led to recovery after a period of several months. Because of the hardness of titanium, drilling of dental inlays should not be attempted! Even if removed, titanium may have migrated into gold inlays and will slowly be released over months or years. I know of two instances where titanium inlays were successfully removed by the use of ultrasonic sound.

Removal of dental amalgam fillings has as yet not been encouraging. Some mercury will remain in the surrounding dental tissue and in various organs in the body. Mercury enters the enterohepatic circulation, often maintaining diarrhea or constipation.

Pleural effusions may require serial thoracocentesis. Pleurodesis relieves pleural effusion but may exacerbate lymphedema of the lower limbs (Kawano et al., 2003). In other patients a pleuroperitoneal (Brofman et al., 1990) or a pleurovenous shunt has been applied (Tanaka et al., 2005).

5.2 Titanium dioxide

Patients taking drugs containing titanium dioxide may have difficulties finding titanium-free replacements. They may have to resort to fluid preparations designed for children, or have titanium-free capsules made. Almost all chewing gums contain titanium dioxide, but not Stimorol senses (except the one with peppermint taste).

6. Summary

Yellow nail syndrome was defined in 1964 to include thick yellow nails and lymphedema. A number of symptoms have later been included, most importantly perhaps sinusitis and chronic cough, because they are easily overlooked by the doctor. Most serious are pleural effusions and protein-losing enteritis. The syndrome is caused by titanium or titanium dioxide.

7. Acknowledgement

All costs for this study were defrayed by the Swedish Society of Dental Amalgam Patients, Trollhättan,Sweden.

8. References

Battaglia A, Di Ricco G, Mariani G & Giuntini C (1985). Pleural effusion and recurrent bronchopneumonia with lymphedema, yellow nails and protein losing enteropathy. *Eur J Respir Dis* 66: 65-69.

Berglund F & Carlmark B (2011). Titanium, sinusitis, and the yellow nail syndrome *Biol Trace Elem Res* 143:1-7.

Böckmann J, Lahl H, Eckert T & Unterhalt B (2000). Titan-Blutspiegel vor und nach Belastungsversuchen mit Titandioxid. *Pharmazie* 55:140-143.

Brofman JD, Hall JB, Scott W & Little AG (1990). Yellow nails, lymphedema and pleural effusion. Treatment of chronic pleural effusion with pleuroperitoneal shunting. 97:743-5

Camilleri AE (1990). Chronic sinusitis and the yellow nail syndrome. *J Laryngol Otol* 104:811–813

Cebeci F, Celebi M & Onsun N (2009). Nonclassical yellow nail syndrome in six-year-old girl: a case report. *Cases J* 2:165–169

D'Allessandro A, Muzi G, Monaco A, Filiberto S, Barboni A & Abbritti G (2001). Yellow nail syndrome: does protein leakage play a role? *Eur Respir J* 17: 149-152.

Danielsson Å, Toth E & Thorlacius H (2006). Capsule endoscopy in the management of a patient with a rare syndrome. *Gut* 55: 196

David-Vaudey E, Jamard B, Hermant C & Cantagrel A (2004). Yellow nail syndrome in rheumatoid arthritis: a drug-induced disease? *Clin Rheumatol* 23: 376-378.

Dilley JJ, Kierland RR, Randall RV & Shick RM (1968). Primary lymphedema associated with yellow nails and pleural effusions. *JAMA* 204:122-125

Duhra PM, Quigley EMM & Marsh MN (1985). Chylous ascites, intestinal lymphoangiectasia and the yellow nail syndrome. *Gut* 26:1266-1269

Emerson PA (1966). Yellow nails, lymphoedema, and pleural effusions. *Thorax* 21: 247-253.

Forsell M, Marcusson JA, Carlmark B & Johansson O (1997). Analysis of the metal content of in vivo fixed dental alloys by means of a simple office procedure. *Swed Dent J* 21: 161-168

Govaert P, Leroy JG, Pauwels R, Vanhaesebrouck P, De Praeter C, Van Kets H & Goeteyn M (1992). Perinatal manifestations of maternal yellow nail syndrome. *Pediatrics* 89:1016-1018

Hassard AD, Martin J & Ross JB (1984). Yellow nail syndrome and chronic sinusitis. *J Otolaryngol* 13:318–320

Hiller E, Rosenow *III* EC & Olsen AM (1972). Pulmonary manifestations of the yellow nail syndrome. *Chest* 61:452-458.

Hunsberger JF (1976). Electrochemical series Table I. In: Weast RC (ed) *Handbook of chemistry and physics*; 57th edn. CRC Press, Boca Raton, pp D141–D143

Jani PU, McCarthy DE & Florence AT (1994). Titanium dioxide (rutile) particle uptake from the rat GI tract and translocation to systemic organs after oral administration. *Int J Pharm* 105: 157-168.

Kawano T, Matsuse H, Shigematsu K, Miyazaki M, Taguchi T & Kohno S (2003). Chemical pleurodesis could exacerbate lymphedema of yellow nail syndrome. *Acta Med Nagasaki* 48:71-72

Malek NP, Ocran K, Tietge UJ, Maschek H, Gratz KF, Trautwein C, Wagner S & Manns MP (1996). A case of the yellow nail syndrome associated with massive chylous ascites, pleural and pericardial effusions. *Z Gastroenterol* 34:763-766.

Müller R-P, Peters PE, Echternacht-Happle K & Happle R (1979). Roentgenographic and clinical signs in yellow nail syndrome. *Lymphology* 12:257-261

Nakielna EM, Wilson J & Ballon HS (1976). Yellow nail syndrome: report of three cases. *Can Med Assoc J* 115:46–48

Reclaru L & Meyer J-M (1998). Effects of fluoride on titanium and other dental alloys in dentistry. *Biomaterials* 19: 85-92

Samman PD & White WF (1964). The "yellow nail" syndrome. *Br J Dermatol* 76:153-157

Schiff N, Grosgogeat B, Lissac M & Dalard F (2002). Influence of fluoride content and pH on the corrosion resistance of titanium and its alloys. *Biomaterials* 23: 1995-2002

Shepherd NA, Crocker PR, Smith AP & Levison DA (1987). Exogenous pigment in Peyer's patches. *Hum Pathol* 18: 50-54.

Slee J, Nelson J, Dickinson J, Kendall P & Halbert A (2000). Yellow nail syndrome presenting as non-immune hydrops: Second case report. *Am J Med Genet* 93:1-4

Strietzel R, Hösch A, Kalbfleisch H, Buch D (1998). In vitro corrosion of titanium. *Biomaterials* 19: 1495-1499.

Tanaka E, Matsumoto K, Shindo T & Taguchi Y (2005). Implantation of a pleurovenous shunt for massive chylothorax in a patient with yellow nail syndrome. *Thorax* 60:254-255.

Varney VA, Cumberworth V, Sudderick R, Durham SR & Mackay IS (1994). Rhinitis, sinusitis and the yellow nail syndrome: a review of symptoms and response to treatment in 17 patients. *Clin Otolaryngol Allied Sci*19:237–240

Wakasa M, Imaizumi T, Suyama A, Takeshita A & Nakamura M (1987) Yellow nail syndrome associated with chronic pericardial effusion. *Chest* 92:366-7.

Wells GC (1966). Yellow nail syndrome with familial primary hypoplasia of lymphatics, manifest late in life. *Proc Royal Soc Med* 59:447

Zerfas AJ (for HJ Wallace). Yellow nail syndrome with bilateral bronchiectasis. *Proc Royal Soc Med* 59: 448.

3

Arm Lymphedema as a Consequence of Breast Cancer Therapy

A. Gabriella Wernicke, Yevgeniya Goltser,
Michael Shamis and Alexander J. Swistel
Weill Cornell Medical College, Department of Radiation Oncology
United States

1. Introduction

Lymphedema is the result of an abnormality of the lymphatic system. It is caused by an excessive accumulation of lymphatic fluid, known as interstitial fluid, in the interstitial tissue, particularly in the subcutaneous fat. Ultimately, this leads to swelling of affected tissues due to a build up of and inadequate lymph drainage, known as lymphedema (Farrow, 2010a) [Figure 1].

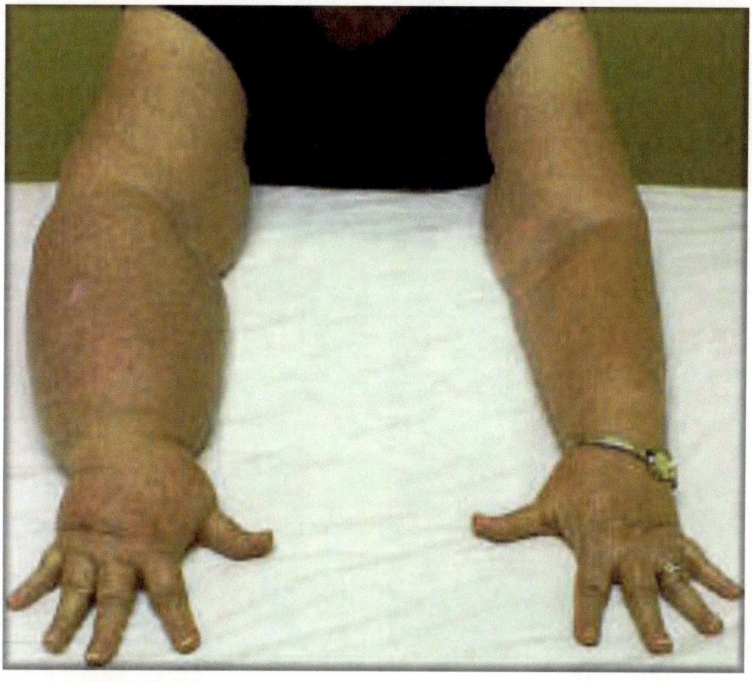

Fig. 1. Right arm lymphedema

Primary lymphedema occurs when people are born with abnormalities in the lymphatic system, such as missing or impaired lymphatic vessels (Farrow, 2010b). The severity of the condition is able to assess whether swelling is present at birth or develops at the onset of puberty or in adulthood. It can affect from one up to four limbs and/or body parts (Farrow, 2010a). Secondary lymphedema is more common and occurs from damage to the lymphatic system that occurs as a result of cancer and its treatment, due to the resection of lymph nodes. Trauma to the skin, such as burns or infections, can also cause secondary lymphedema (Gordon, 2007; Piller, 2009).

Signs and symptoms of progressive lymphedema include discomfort and pain associated with full sensation in the limb(s) and the skin feeling tight, as well as difficulty with daily tasks due to a decreased flexibility in the hand, wrist, or ankle and the inability to fit into clothing and jewelry in a certain area. Progressive lymphedema is complicated by recurrent infections, non-healing wounds, as well as emotional and social distress (Ridner, 2009; Ahmed, 2008; Shih, 2009).

Lymphedema is prevalent and most often studied as a consequence of breast cancer. However, it has been studied in cases of melanoma, gynecological cancer, head and neck cancer as well as sarcoma (Lewin et al., 2010; Murphy et al., 2010; Smith et al., 2010; Cormier et al., 2010; Lacomba, 2010). Research shows that there is a lifelong risk of developing lymphedema due to cancer and the overall risk has been reported to be 15.5% (Chang et al., 2010) [Figure 2].

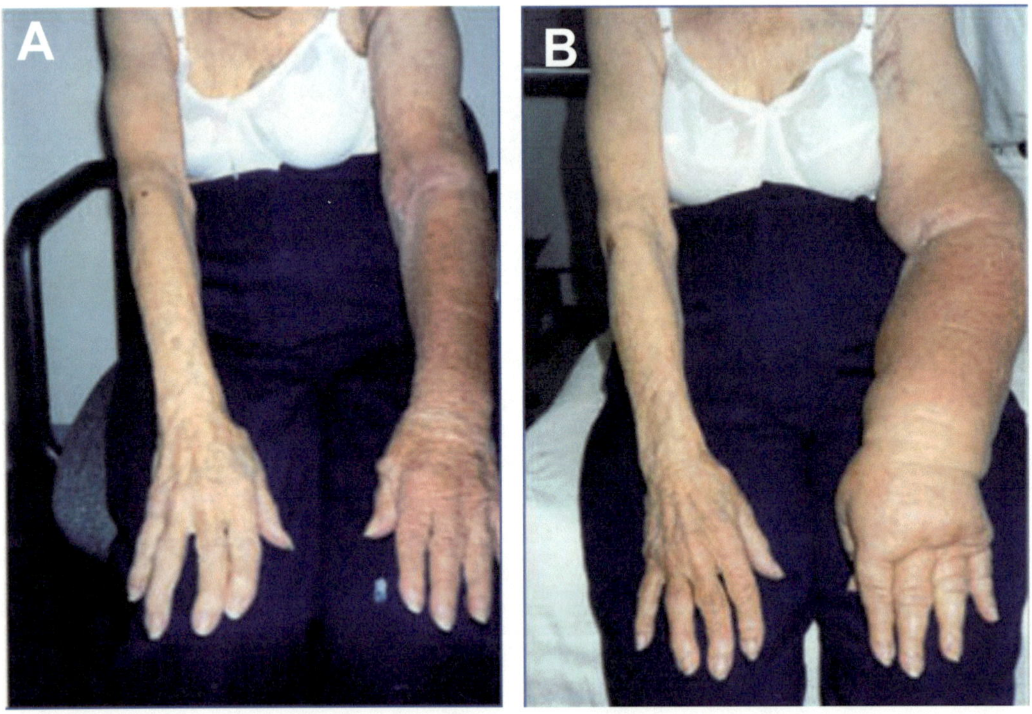

Fig. 2. A woman with locally advanced breast cancer status post left modified radical mastectomy and lymph node dissection and radiotherapy to the left chest wall, supraclavicular area and axillary lymph nodes. **A.** Left arm at 3 months after treatment. **B.** Left arm demonstrates marked lymphedema at 3 years after treatment.

Both primary and secondary lymphedemas possess characteristic features that can be distinguished over time. History should include information such as age of onset, location(s) of swelling, pain and other symptoms of discomfort, medications that instigate swelling, the course of progression of swelling, and factors prompting swelling such as cancer, injury, or infection. Family history is important to diagnose inherited forms of lymphedema (Gupta, 2006). A physical examination assesses the vascular system, the soft tissue and skin surrounding the swollen body parts, palpation of lymph nodes, and looks for changes in the body systems in accordance with inherited lymphedemas (Wang, 2005; Moseley et al., 2008). Further diagnostic tests and imagining coupled with history, family history, and physical examination are used to correctly diagnose a patient (Lewin et al., 2010; Smith et al., 2010).

Lympehedema is a type of side effect requiring attention to diagnosis and management by a number of specialists taking care of a patient with breast cancer. It is critical for each discipline to pay particular attention to the patients' subjective reporting of their symptoms suggestive of lymphedema. Therefore, a multidisciplinary approach to diagnosis and management of lympehedema is essential for the routine surveillance after treatment by all the involved physicians, including the surgeon, radiation oncologist, and medical oncologist. A lymphedema specialist's consultation is often necessary, especially when the patient is at risk for developing lymphedema or has an evidence of this diagnosis on physical examination.

2. Diagnosis of lymphedema

Physical examination includes placing hands on location of lymphedema and feeling palpation as well as the surrounding area of the affected limb. This procedure is called subjective palpation. Upon physical examination, the standard way of detecting lymphedema is by taking measures of limb volume (Chen et al., 2008; Cheville et al., 2003; Hayes et al., 2005). An enlargement, or increase in volume, of the limb is the result of fluid build up in the tissues. Volume is measured by 3 methods including tape measurements, perometry, and water displacement. These measurements of volume illustrate the presence and severity of the condition (Unno et al., 2008). Tape measurements are most accurate when done at precisely defined intervals and when taken by the same individual, ultimately using geometric formulas to determine the total volume.

Perometry uses an infra-red optical electronic scanner to calculate volume by precisely positioning the body part exactly the same each time and calibrating the machine (Rockson et al., 2007). This method can detect volume changes in breast cancer survivors as little as 3% (Czerneic et al., 2010). Water displacement measurements are taken by immersing the limb in a large cylinder and determining the volume of water displaced, or pushed out of the cylinder. However, measuring volume cannot differentiate lymphedema from other types of edema and is a technique best used as follow up for treatment of lymphedema rather then diagnosis (Unno et al., 2008).

A radiological technique, that detects slow or absent lymph flow and areas of reflux or backup of lymph node and lymph vessel imaging due to lymphedema is called a lymphoscintigraphy. Normally, technetium labeled sulfur is the radio-labeled particle of protein injected directly under the skin to detect and image the affected area (Piller, 2009; Szuba et al., 2003; Hayes et al., 2008; Bellini et al., 2005). The procedure identifies lymphatic problems at late stages of lymphedema and shows the basics of the peripheral lymphatic system and larger more prominent lymph nodes and vessels. Radiology dpartments are apt at performing lymphoscintigraphy studies aimed at identifying the sentinel lymph node for cancers of the breast and ultimately further studies for the diagnosis of lymphedema Cornish et al., 2007; Szuba et al., 2000, 2003, 2007)

A more recent technique of lymph vessel imaging uses indocyanine green (ICG) injections into the skin and an infrared fluorescence camera to detect the function of even the smallest lymphatic vessels. This is called Near Infra-Red Florescence Imaging (NIR). NIR-ICG can pick up early stages of lymphedema and diagnose diseased non-contracting lymphatics even before swelling occurs (Farrow, 2010; Adams et al.; Rasmussen et al., 2009, 2010; Unno et al., 2010; Maus, 2010)

There is a variety of diagnostic tests that can be performed in order to classify and detect lymphedema. These include soft tissue imaging, bioimpedance spectroscopy, tonometry, genetic testing, various forms of vascular imaging, as well as blood tests (Farrow, 2010).

Soft tissue imaging like MRIs (magnetic resonance imaging), CTs (computed tomography scans, and US (ultrasounds) detect excess fluid in the tissues. Since lymphedema is the result of interstitial fluid build up these imaging techniques are often used to determine the cause of the condition as well as lymphedema that is a result of an untreated cancer (Astrom et al., 2001; Deltombe et al., 2007; Unno et al., 2008)

Bioimpedance Spectroscopy (BIS) measures water content in tissues by passing a small, harmless, electrical current through the limb in order to measure the impedance to current flow. The higher the water content in the area the lower the resistance. BIS assesses the condition by comparing the resistance of electrical flow in the intracellular and interstitial fluid of a whole limb, because calculations are performed to the length of the body part (Gergich et al., 2008; Ward, 2006; Rockson et al., 2007).

Lymphedema is graded according to increased size as well as staging of the progression in the change of the skin texture. As a consequence lymphedema the skin and subcutaneous tissue become harder and denser (Executive Committee of International Society of Lymphology, 2009). Upon physical examination, tissue texture, pitting, larger skin folds, wounds or papillomas are noted. Current examinations to determine skin texture and resistance are tissue dielectric constant and tonometry. The tissue dielectric constant measures tissue water content and uses a specific frequency of an electrical current to measure the reflected return wave in order to indicate how much water is present in the tissue (Mayrovitz, 2009; Corica et al., 2006; Mirnajafi et al., 2004; Ridner et al., 2007). Tonometry determines how firm a tissue is by measuring how much force is needed to indent the tissue sample (Mayrovitz, 2009) [Figure 3].

Young patients diagnosed with primary lymphedema should undergo genetic testing and counseling and have a karyotype test performed in order to detect abnormalities. Turner's syndrome has been linked to lymphedema and can be determined from a karyotype. Specific genes are also associated with lymphedema (Ferrell, 2008). These include FOXC2 an SOX18 (Connell et al., 2009; Brice et al, 2002). However, inherited lymphedema is not detectible on gene or chromosome tests and genetic testing for late-onset lymphedema does not prove to have benefits (Farrow, 2010b).

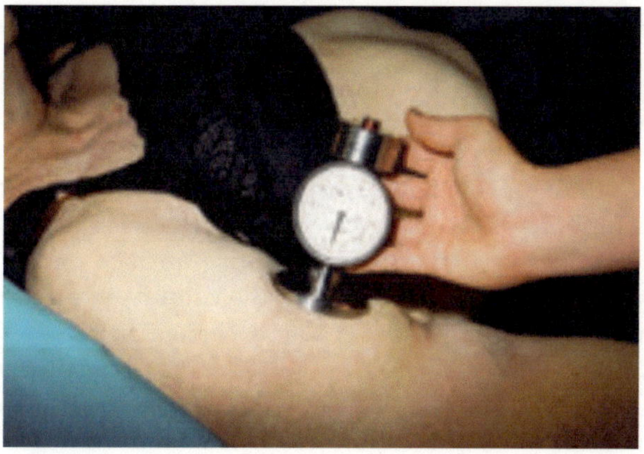

Fig. 3. A tonometer is used to assess the firmness of a tissue by measuring how much force is needed to indent the tissue sample.

Cardiovascular diseases or abnormalities may also serve as a trigger for many forms of edema (Schumacher et al., 2008). For those given a diagnosis of primary lymphedema, it is important to determine if congestive heart failure, deep venous thrombosis, damaged valves in the vein or any arterial conditions account for the swelling or are an adjunct to existent lymphedema (Szuba, 2000; Bellini, 2005). Secondary lymphedema, as a result of cancer, can be studied by taking images of the heart, veins and valves to determine the case, severity, and treatment options of the edema. Cardiovascular studies usually ordered for edema studies include echocardiogram, venous ultrasound, and arterial ultrasound with ankle brachial index (ABI). It is best to do ultrasounds in a standing up position to test for incompetency of the valves. More advanced forms of imaging for insufficiency of blood vessels is by means of a computed tomography, venogram, and arteiogram. These are normally used to assess conditions in the chest, abdomen, or pelvis (Farrow, 2010).

Blood tests are unavailable for diagnosis of lymphedema. However, conditions that mimic lymphedema's symptoms such as hypothyroidism or hypoproteinemia may cause swelling and need to be assessed by means of a blood test. For some lymphedemas that are genetically inherited x-rays are important to detect orthopedic abnormalities (Bellini et al., 2009; Gupta et al., 2006).

3. Lymphedema as a long-term sequelae of breast cancer therapy

There are recommended guidelines to follow for optimal prevention, screening and measurement for early detection of breast cancer related lymphedema (Farrow, 2010c). There should be a pro-active approach pre-operatively and post-operatively for arm measurements taken by patients and physicians. Patients should receive risk-reduction strategies prior to treatment (NLN Position Paper, 2011; Fu et al., 2010). Weight and height should be accurately measured during each visit to a specialist in order to determine body mass index (BMI). A BMI greater than or equal to 25 warrants a consultation with a dietician and a BMI greater or equal to 30 warrants a consultation with a dietician and a weight reduction (Ridner et al., 2011; Helyer et al., 2010; Centers for Disease Control, 2011).

Patients that have been diagnosed with breast cancer should have baseline pre and post-treatment arm measurements taken on both arms and should be given this information to share with other healthcare providers. Lymphedema warrants active surveillance post-treatment for such symptoms as swelling, heaviness or tightness in the affected arm(s), and at-risk chest and truncal areas. If there appears to be an increase of 1 cm in any of the circumference measurements when compared to the contralateral limb, the patient should schedule a follow-up visit in 1 month. A 2 cm change in any of the circumferential measurements or a 5% volume change in an at-risk limb warrant immediate referral for further evaluation by a professional trained in lymphedema assessment and management. Subjective symptom reports should be taken seriously and may include perceived swelling, tightness, tingling, and heaviness (Farrow, 2010c).

Surgical techniques of managing breast cancer and long-term morbidity include radical mastectomy, modified radical mastectomy, and lumpectomy. Surgical approaches to axillary treatment include sentinel lymph node dissection (SLND) and axillary lymph node dissection (ALND). The number of lymph nodes that defines ALND is 10, and the standard ALND involved at least dissection of levels I-II axillary lymph nodes, based on the arbitrarily set anatomic Berg principles (Berg, 1955). Identification of a sentinel lymph node for SLND is typically done by either an injection of the isosulfan blue dye, the technetium (99mTc)-sulphur colloid, or both. All blue-stained nodes and/or nodes with radioactive counts, as measured with the gamma probe, are defined as sentinel lymph nodes. Typically, the number of nodes sample as a result of a SLND is small, with a median number of 2 nodes (Wernicke, 2010).

A number of efforts have been employed to minimize the risk of lymphedema (Figure 2B), as it is associated with the dissection of a large number of axillary lymph nodes. Various studies have determined the incidence of lymphedema depending on the type of lymph node dissection, ALND versus SLND. Table I summarizes the incidence of lymphedema based on the type of axillary lymph node surgery – SLND or ALND – from a number of published studies for both node negative and node positive patients. The Milan trial, the Sentinella/GIVOM trial, The ALMANAC-UK trial, and the NSABP B-32 trial all showcase node negative patients in the varying prospective randomized trials (Veronesi et al., 2003, 1997; Land et al., 2010; Mclaughlin et al., 2008; Ashikaga et al., 2008; Mansel et al., 2006). In the Milan Trial, at the median follow up of 3 years lymphedema, as assessed by a medical professional, was detectable in 7/100 (7%) of patients in the SLND group in contrast with 75/100 (75%) of cases of lymphedema in the ALND group (Veronesi et al., 2003, 1997). In the Sentinella/GIVOM trial, it was found that the odds ratio of sentinel lymph node to axillary lymph node was 0.52 at their median follow up of 4.6 years (Land et al., 2010). In the ALMANAC-UK trial, with a short median follow up of 1 year lymphedema was assessed by a patient and was reported in 20/412 (4.9%) of patients in the SLND group in contrast with 53/403 (13%) of cases of lymphedema in the ALND group (Mclaughlin et al., 2008).

Published studies	Median follow up (years)	N	Inclusion Criteria	Lymphedema by medical professionals (%)	Lymphedema by patients (%)
MILAN (Veronesi et al., 1997, 2003) (negative SLN in 341patients (167SLN +174ALND) (1998-1999)	3	516	<2cm, L only (wide excision or quadran-tectomy)	* 7/100 (7) # 75/100 (75)	N/A
Sentinella/ GIVOM (Land et al., 2010) (1999-2004)	4.6	749	<3cm, L,MRM	0.52[2]	N/A
ALMANAC-UK (Mclaughlin et al., 2008) (1999-2003)	1	1031	<2, 2-5,>5cm, L, MRM, axillary RT	N/A	* 20/412 (5)[1] # 53/403 (13)[1]
ACOSZOG Z0011 Trial (Aareleid et al., 2002) (1999-2004)	3	891	<2cm, L, with 1-2 +SLN	* 14/226 (6) # 26/242 (11)	* 14/253 (5) # 52/272 (19)
NSABP B-32 Morbidty results (Ashikaga et al., 2010) (1999-2004)	3	5611	≤2.0, 2.1-4.0, >4.0 cm, L or M	*303/1459 (20.8) # 431/1421 (30.3)	N/A
NSABP B-32 Outcome study (Mansel et al., 2006) (2001-2004)	3	749	≤2.0, 2.1-4.0, ≥4.1 cm, L or M	N/A	*10/320 (3) # 25/307 (8)
Wernicke et al. (Wernicke et al., 2010, 2011)	10	265	<5.0cm, L	*6/111 (5.4) #21/115 (18.3)	* 10/111 (10.0) # 39/115 (33.9)

L=lumpectomy
MRM=modified radical mastectomy
RT=radiotherapy
*SLND=Sentinel Lymph Node
SLN +ALN=Sentinel Lymph Node+Axillary Lymph Node
[1] Summation of patients with mild and severe symptoms.
[2] Odds ratio (SLN/ALN)

Table 1. A summary of incidence of lymphedema from the published studies.

In the NSABP B-32 trial, at a 3-year follow-up lymphedema was assessed by both medical professionals and by patients themselves. When assessed by the former, the incidence of lymphedema was 303/1459 (20.8%) of patients in the SLND group in contrast with 431/1421 (30.3%) of cases of lymphedema in the ALND group. However, the patient self-assessment group demonstrated the rate of lymphedema as 10/320 (3.1%) in the SLND cohort and occurred in 25/307 (8.1%) of women in the ALND group (Ashikaga et al., 2008; Mansel et al., 2006). One of the largest retrospective reviews of a mature 10-year follow-up of experience from Thomas Jefferson University Hospital conducted by Wernicke et al, also assessed lymphedema by two methodologies. It was evident that regardless of whether the assessment was performed by a medical professional or a patient, there was statistically significant difference in the rates of this complication between the two cohorts as experienced by patients. When assessed by a medical professional, lymphedema was detectable in 6/111 (5.4%) of patients in the SLND group in contrast with 21/115 (18.3%) of cases of lymphedema in the ALND group, respectively ($p<0.0001$). The patient self-assessment groups demonstrated the lymphedema in 10/111 (10.0%) of patients in the SLND cohort and 39/115 (33.9%) of women reporting this complication in the ALND group ($p<0.0001$). This difference appears to be sustainable even a decade after the surgery, and the percentage of patients that experienced chronic lymphedema is significantly greater in the ALND cohort as compared with the SLND one (Wernicke et al., 2010) [Table 1].

The ACOSOG Z001 trial assessed patients with clinically positive axillary nodes (Aareleid et al. 2002). In this study, lymphedema was also assessed by the dual methodologies of a medical professional and a patient self-assessment. At a median follow-up age of 3 years, when assessed by a medical professional, lymphedema was detected in 14/226 (6%) of patients in the SLND group in contrast with 26/242 (11%) of cases of lymphedema in the ALND group. The patient self-assessment groups demonstrated the incidence of lymphedema in 14/253 (5%) of patients in the SLND cohort and 52/272 (19%) of women reporting this complication in the ALND group [Table I].

Could radiotherapy be a contributing factor to the complications of axillary surgery? If a low incidence of ALN failures lies in sterilization of the occult metastases in the axillary lymph nodes with the conventional breast tangential ports delivering RT to a patient in a supine position (Wernicke et al., 2010), radiotherapy may be at least in part responsible for the morbidity attributable to surgery. Goodman et al reported that with the standard radiation tangents, 90% of the Berg level I axilla and up to 70% of level II axillary lymph nodes received 95% of the prescribed dose to the breast (Smitt et al., 1999). Figure 4 demonstrates a typical patient treated with 3-D radiotherapy in the supine position with the standard tangential radiation fields targeting the breast tissue and inadvertently providing at least partial coverage for at least two of the Berg axillary levels. The vast majority of literature, with only a few negative studies, supports the fact that the modern 3-D tangential radiation port of the breast, administered in supine position, will at least partially irradiate the undissected axillary lymph nodes stations (Smitt et al., 1999; Takeda et al., 2000, 2004; Krasin et al., 2000; Aristei et al., 2001; Schlembach et al., 2001; **Orecchia et al., 2005;** Wong et al., 2008; Rabinovitch et al., 2008). This phenomenon may explain why even patients with SLND experience lymphedema as a long-term toxicity [Wernicke et al., 2010].

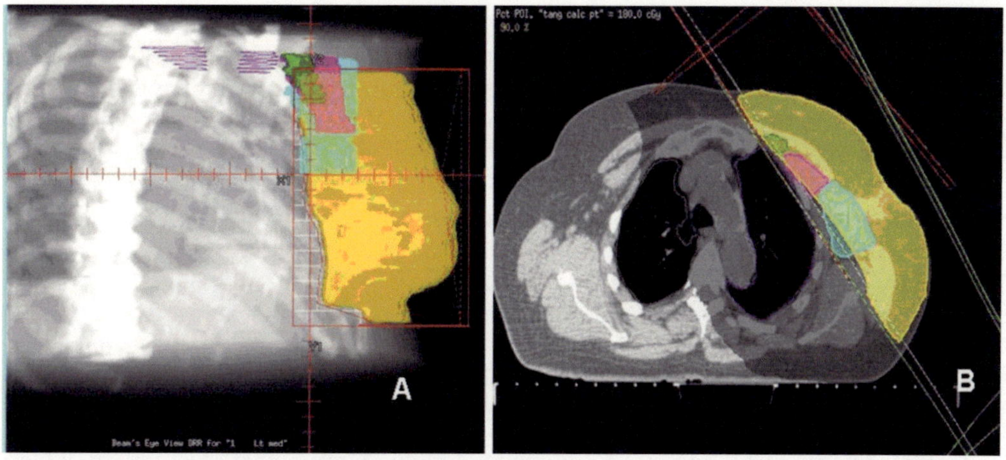

Fig. 4. **A.** A relationship between local breast tangent radiation field and regional lymph nodes as depicted in the lateral beam's eye view with a tangential portal, where the superior border of the radiation portal is set below the heads of the clavicles (navy). **B.** The axial image through the dissected axilla demonstrates Level I (blue), Level II (purple), and Level III (dark green) axillary lymph nodal stations which are partially covered by the 90% isodose area covering the breast tissue (orange).

Does lymphedema have any risks associated with the use of systemic therapy? No significantly increased risk of incidence of lymphedema was observed in the literature with systemic therapy using hormonal treatment (Norman et al., 2010). Chemotherapy has been reported in some series to increase the complication rate associated with breast RT, including arm edema (Meek, 1998). However, no formal studies report any concrete data, which can predict such outcomes.

4. Treatment of lymphedema

4.1 Non-invasive management techniques

The main, "gold standard" of treatment for lymphedema is Combined, Complex or Comprehensive Decongestive Therapy (CDT) (Mayrovitz, 2009). The initial reductive phase of CDT treatment is known as Phase I. The main goals are to reduce the size of the affected location and to improve the skin. Phase II is known as the maintenance phase, where the patient self-manages to keep the effects of phase I treatment long term (Szuba, 2000; Hinrichs et al., 2004; Lasinski, 2002; Thomas et al., 2007; Koul et al., 2007). The effects of CDT include decreases in swelling, an increase in lymph drainage from the congested areas, a reduction in skin fibrosis and improvements in the skin conditions, an enhancement in the patient's functional status and quality of life as well as a relief in discomfort, and a reduced risk of cellulitis and Steward-Treves-Syndrome (a rare form of angiosarcoma) (Hammer et al., 2007; Mondry et al., 2004; Ferrandez, 1996; Franzcek et al., 1997; Hayes et al., 2008; Ahmed, 2008; Weiss, 2002; Kim et al., 2007; Cormier et al., 2009; Hormes et al., 2010; Fu et al., 2009; Vignes, 2006).

Components of Combined, Complex or Comprehensive Decongestive Therapy include manual lymph drainage (MLD), multi-layer, short-stretch compression bandaging, lymphatic exercise, skin care, and education in lymphedema management as well as elastic compression garments (Didem et al., 2005; Ko, 1998). There are to phases of CDT: Phase I (Reductive) and Phase II (Maintenance). The first phase's frequency and duration should be altered as to produce the best possible outcome of improvements in skin and reduction in swelling of the affected area in the shortest time period. Normally, CDT is completed within 3 to 8 weeks and administered daily, or 5 days per week (Mayrovitz, 2009; Ko, 1998; Yamamoto et al., 2008). The second phase of CDT is a self-management program is set up directly following completion of phase I. It includes self-lymph drainage, home lymphatic exercises, a skin regimen, and self-application of compression garments or bandages (Yamamoto, 2008). Phase II must be monitored and changed periodically to ensure effectiveness. This includes changing compression garments every 4-6 months and equipment replacements and maintenance. Monitoring by a medical profession is, also, essential to the long-term success for lymphedema treatment (Ko, 1998; Hafner et al., 2005; Boris et al., 1994; Johnstone et al., 2006; Lasinski, 2002).

Therapists providing CDT care are recommended by the Lymphology Association of North America® (LANA®) to have a minimum of 135 hours of training. Additional training may be required for specialists treating facial, truncal, and genital lymphedema and patients with complex diseases or illnesses (Farrow, 2010b; Czerneic et al., 2010).

Manual lymph drainage is a manual, hands-on, part of CDT care that prompts superficial lymphatic vessels to remove excess interstitial fluid which is then moved through the subepidermal fluid channels formed as a result of damage of the lymphatics (Williams et al., 2002). Certified Lymphedema therapists use the MLD technique to stimulate fluid removal from areas where the lymphatics are not working properly into working lymph vessels and nodes (McNeely, 2004).

Compression bandaging creates gradient compression by effectively utilizing multiple layers of several materials. Components of compression bandaging include tubular bandage lining, digit bandages, polyester, cotton, or foam under-cast padding, and multiple layers of short-stretch bandages with 50% overlap and 50% stretch to cover the entire limb. Short-stretch bandages stretch to 40-60% from resting length and long-stretch bandages stretch to greater than 140% of resting length. Short-stretch bandages are applied with low to moderate tension and are more prominent at the ends of extremities, reduce tissue hardening, also known as fibrosis (Farrow, 2010b; Brice et al., 2002; King, 2001; Williams, 2005; Lerner, 2000; Foldi et al., 2005)

Exercise, including lymphatic "Remedial Exercise", has been shown to have increased beneficial effects for patients with lymphedema. Patients are encouraged to create individualized exercise programs with a lymphedema specialist (Schmitz et al., 2009; Johansson et al., 2005; Mustian et al., 2009). Exercise must be done while wearing a compression garment or bandage to alleviate the build up of interstitial fluid (Gultig, 2005).

Hygiene is an important factor in lymphedema treatment which aides in reducing the amount of fungus and bacteria present on the skin. Cracks and dry skin are entry points for these pathogens and it is recommended that patients use low pH moisturizers to hydrate the skin and alleviate drying and cracking, which can lead to infections and wounds (Vaillant, 2002; Mallon, 1994). Typical infection of the skin is known as cellulitis and, ultimately, requires antibiotic treatment in people with lymphedema (Czerneic et al., 2010; Al Niaimi et al., 2009; Cooper et al., 2009; Godoy et al., 2007).

After maximal volume reduction in Phase I CDT, patients will be fitted to any one of the following compression garments, depending on the affected body part: sleeves, stockings, bras, compression shorts, or face and neck compression wear. The patient will receive two compression garments one to wear and one to wash and dry. This is done to prevent wearing dirty or wet compression wear, which will promote growth of fungus and bacteria. Garments should be washed daily and replaced every 4-6 months to maintain the same compression strength. It is important the garment be properly fitted to the proper garment style and compression strength to maintain long-term control of the lymphedema in terms of volume control and skin health. Custom garments are made for those patients who cannot fit into ready-made garments and allow for special options such as reduction of risk of breakdown of skin or fastening devices for easier removal or putting on of the garment. There are both day and night or advanced day garments (Yasuhara, 1996; Badger et al., 2000; Cornu-Thenard et al., 2007). The latter come in specialized varieties that better help to maintain the results of Phase I CDT, throughout Phase II. These include Velcro closure and specialized foam compression garments (Lund, 2000; Hafner et al., 2005; Lawrence, 2008).

Seeing that lymphedema is a life-long condition, maintenance is very important (Fu et al., 2008). Self-care includes education on risk-reduction practices, self-lymph drainage, skin care, signs and symptoms of infection, proper fit and care of garments, and the importance of good nutrition, as well as healthy regiments of exercise and weight control (Farrow, 2010b). The risk of getting lymphedema increases with obesity. Therefore, it is important to maintain or lose to be at a normal, healthy weight (Gur et al., 2009; Petrek, 2001; Soran et al., 2006; Helyer et al., 2010). It has been proven that the arm volume of post-mastectomy lymphedema patients decreases in overweight patients with weight loss (Shaw et al., 2007). Other patient conditions, such as scars, musculoskeletal ailments, palliative care necessities, post-radiation fibrosis, may require alterations in the CDT program. Adaptations are additions to CDT and include therapy, scar massage or myofacial therapy (Lund, 2000; Mallon, 1994; Yamamoto et al., 2008)

Compression pump therapy or Intermittent Pneumatic Compression Therapy (IPC) can be used as either an adjunct to Phase I CDT or as a component of Phase II CDT. These pumps should have a individualized pattern of a multi-chamber system that stimulates lymph flow in a single direction based on the pattern and diagnosis of lymphedema. Since lymphedema is a result of a condition in a quadrant of the body as well as the limb, the pump must work to treat the condition as a whole (Shaw et al., 2007; Miranda et al., 2001; Yamazaki, 1988; Dini, 1998; Partsch, 1980; Hammond et al., 2009; Ridner et al., 2008; Szolnoky et al., 2009). Normal pump pressures range between 30-60 mmHg (Olszewski, 2009). Recent studies show possible false correlations between the skin and device interface pressure patterns. This may have an ultimate effect on therapy (Mayrovitz, 2007). Higher pressures are more dangerous because they may do harm to superficial structures (Segers et al., 2002). The length of treatment is normally 1 hour (Hammond et al., 2009; Ridner et al., 2008).

Patients considered for IPC therapy need to be evaluated by a physician with medical knowledge of lymphedema. The evaluation provides level of pain and skin sensitivity as well as pressure for application to fibrotic areas. With trunk, chest or genital swelling is present, the physician must determine whether a pump that provides appliances to treat those areas is necessary or if the patient can manage the trunk swelling through self-MLD or garments. If a pump with only extremity attachments used, monitoring of a condition known as fibroscelerotic ring should be a must, to detect an increase in hardening of the tissue or edema above the device sleeve (Boris, 1998). If this occurs both the extremities and the trunk should be treated (Olszewski, 2009, Brice et al. 2002).

IPC should not be administered with the following conditions: acute infection, severe arterial vascular disease, acute superficial or deep vein phlebitis (inflammation or clot), recurrent cancer in the affected area, or uncompensated congestive heart failure (Farrow, 2010b).

5. Invasive management techniques

Surgical treatment for lymphedema is performed under special circumstances, when the condition's severity supersedes all possible treatment options to control it, and in unison with CDT. Surgery has been used to reduce the weight of that part of the body that suffers from the condition, minimize the recurring inflammatory attacks, improve aesthetics, and to fit the limb into garments (Gloviczki, 1999; Vignes, 2002). Several surgical options have proven to work on lymphedema patients including debulking and liposuction, tissue transfers and microsurgical lymphatic reconstruction. Debulking surgery aims at removing hard connective tissue as well as large folds of fatty tissue that presents as a consequence of the condition. After this operation patients must wear compression garments to maintain the after effects of surgery, which include lymphatic scarring and lymphatic insufficiency. However, prolonged hospitalizations, poor healing of wounds, nerve damage or loss, intense scarring, negative effects on lymphatic vessels in that limb's area, aesthetically displeasing results, and even loss of function in the limb may occur (Farrow, 2010b; Miller, 1998; Salgado et al., 20009; Kim, 2004).

Liposuction, performed under general anesthesia, is the removal of fatty tissue deposits and the creation of many small incisions in the affected body part withstanding a long history with the lymphedema condition. The fat is suctioned out by means of tubular suction devices which breaks up and liquefies it. Tight bandaging is necessary post surgery to stop bleeding and compression garments are worn life-long to prevent lymphedema recurrence due to possible scarring of the lymph vessels during the procedure. Bleeding, infection, skin loss, unordinary sensations, and recurrence may occur post-operatively (Brorson, 2003; Brorson et al., 2006; Fazhi et al., 2009). Tissue grafts, or tissue transfers, are less well known forms of surgery for effectively treating lymphedema. Their overall goal is to bring lymph vessels into congested areas for better removal of excess interstitial fluid (Fazhi et al., 2009; Slavin et al., 1999)

Microsurgical and supramicrosurgical treatments, similarly aim at draining excess lymphatic fluid by means of shuttling lymph vessels to more congested areas. Although no long-term studies have been conducted on the effectiveness of this surgery, there have been limb volume reductions and successful connections of lymph vessels and veins, lymph nodes and veins, and multiple lymph vessels (Weiss et al., 2003; Becker et al., 2006; Baumeister, 2003a, 2003b; Koshima, 2000; Chang, 2010; Campisi et al., 2006). Surgical treatment of affected lymphedema sights is risky and very rarely a necessary consideration. If surgical treatment is considered, CDT is still a necessary adjunct and compression garments and Phase II maintenance is crucial (Warren et al., 2007).

6. Pharmacological, complementary integrative and alternative management

Pharmaceutical approaches to lymphedema have shown that treatment with drugs, such as Diosmin and Coumarin, or dietary supplements alone is ineffective. Diuretics cannot effectively remove interstitial fluid from the tissues, but may ultimately result in dehydration, electrolyte imbalance, or tissue damage. However patients with a history of hypertension and cardiovascular disease should speak to a healthcare provider or doctor before stopping use of diuretics (Farrow, 2010b; Loprinzi, 1999; Taylor, 1993; Cotonat, 1989).

Little research from studies has proved that all natural supplements are beneficial for lymphedema patients. Selenium has been proven to aide in lymphedema as a consequence of head and neck cancers. However, bromelain and American horse chestnut have not been studied for lymphedema related specific cases. Any natural supplements should be discussed with a physician prior to ingestion (Siebert et al., 2002; Micke et al., 2003; Bruns et al., 2004; Cirelli, 1962; Kelly, 1996; Gaby, 1995).

Ongoing research has been presented in treatments such as cold laser, electrical stimulation, vibratory therapy, oscillation therapy, endermologie and aqualymphatic therapy and are done in combination with portions of CDT (Piller et al., 2010; Carati et al., 2003; Hafner et al., 2005; Lawrence, 2008; Tidhar et al., 201; Omar et al., 2010; Jahr, et al., 2008). Acupuncture is shown to ease some cancer and treatment related symptoms such as fatigue, hot flashes, nausea, neuropathy, and muscular or joint pain, but no formal treatment has been devised from acupuncture (Farrow, 2010b).

7. Conclusions

Overall, lymphedema is a serious condition that requires timely intervention and appropriate therapy. The multidisciplinary approach is important to a patient at risk for lymphedema. It is important that early education on lymphedema be a standard of management and care for all patients. Prevention, screening, and measurement are all important for early detection of breast cancer related lymphedema. The conservative surgical approach minimizes a breast cancer patient's long-term risk of lymphedema, as does hormonal therapy. Chemotherapy, on the other hand, may have risks associated with developing lymphedema after breast cancer.

8. References

Aareleid T, Brenner H. Trends in cancer patient survival in Estonia before and after the transition from a Soviet Republic to an open-market economy. *Int. J. Cancer.* 2002; 102, 45–50.

Adams,KE et al. Direct Evidence of lymphatic function improvement after advanced pneumatic compression device treatment of lymphedema. Biomedical Optics Express 1, 114

Ahmed, R. J (2008) Lymphedema and Quality of Life in Breast Cancer. Survivors: The Iowa Women's Health Study. Clin Oncol 26, 5689-5696

Al Niaimi, F et al. (2009) Cellulitis and Lymphoedema, A Vicious Cycle. Journal of Lymphoedema. 4, 38-42

Aristei C, Chionne F, Marsella A, Alessandro M, Rulli A, Lemmi A, Perrucci E, Latini P. Evaluation of level I and II axillary nodes included in the standard breast tangential fields and calculation of the administered dose: results of a prospective study. *Int J Radiat Oncol Biol Phys*2001;51:69–73.

Ashikaga T, Krag D, Land S, Julian T, Anderson S, Brown A, Skelly J, Harlow S, Weaver D, Mamounas E, Costantino J, Wolmark N. Morbidity results from the NSABP B-32 trial comparing sentinel lymph node dissection versus axiallary dissection. *J. Surg. Oncol.* 2010;102:111–118.

Astrom K et al.(2001) Imaging of primary, secondary and mixed forms of lymphedema. Acta Radiol. 42 409-416

Badger CM, et al (2000) A randomized, controlled, parallel-group clinical trial comparing multilayer bandaging followed by hosiery versus hosiery alone in the treatment of patients with lymphedema of the limb. Cancer 88, 2832-37

Baumeister, R.G. (2003). The microsurgical lymph vessel transplantation. Handchir Mikrochir Plast Chir, 35, 202-209.

Becker C, et al (2006) Post mastectomy lymphedema: long-term results following microsurgical lymph node transplantation. Ann Surg; 243, 313-315)

Bellini C. (2005) Pulmonary Lymphangiectasia. 38, 111-121

Bellini C et al (2005) Diagnostic Protocol for Lymphoscintigraphy in Newborns. Lymphology 38, 9-15

Bellini C et al. (2009) Congenital lymphatic dysplasias: genetics review and resources for the lymphologist. Lymphology 42, 36-41

Berg JW. The significance of axillary node levels in the study of breast carcinoma. **Cancer.** 1955;8(4):776-778.

Boris, M. (1998). The risks of genital lymphedema after pump treatment for lower limb lymphedema. Lymphology. 31. 50-20.

Boris M, et al (1994). Lymphedema reduction by noninvasive complex lymphedema therapy. Oncology. 9, 95-106

Brice, G et al (2002) Analysis of the phenotypic abnormalities in lymphoedema- distichiasis syndrome in 74 patients with FOXC2 mutations or linkage to 16q24. J Med Genet, 39, 478-483.

Brorson, H. (2003). Liposuction in arm lymphedema treatment. Scand J Surg. 92, 287-95.

Brorson H, Ohlin K, Olsson G, Svensson B. Liposuction of leg lymphedema: Preliminary 2 year results. Lymphology 2006; 39

Bruns F, et al.(2004) Selenium in the treatment of head and neck lymphedema. Med. Princ Pract. 13:185-90.

Campisi C, et al, (2006) Lymphatic microsurgery for the treatment of lymphedema. Microsurgery; 26(1): 65-69.

Carati C, et al. Treatment of Postmastectomy Lymphedema with Low-Level Laser Therapy. Cancer 2003;98:1114–22

Centers for Disease Control. (2011). About BMI for adults.

http://www.cdc.gov/healthyweight/assessing/bmi/adult_bmi/index.html

Cormier, JN et al. (2009) Minimal limb volume change has a significant impact on breast cancer survivors. Lymphology 42, 161-175

Cornish, B et al. (2007) Can bioimpedance spectroscopy tell us about the form of lymphoedema? In Scharfetter and Merwa (Eds) 13th International Conference on

Electrical Bioimpedance and 8th Conference on Bioimpedance Tomography. Springer. 795-798.

Czerneic, S et al (2010) Segmental measurement of breast cancer-related arm lymphoedema using perometry and bioimpedance spectroscopy. Support Care Cancer. Online DOI: 10.1007/s00520-010-0896-8

Chang, D. (2010): Lymphaticovenular Bypass for Lymphedema Management in Breast Cancer Patients: A Prospective Study. Plastic & Reconstructive Surgery 126, 752-758.

Chang, S et al (2010) Prospective assessment of postoperative complications and associated costs following inguinal lymph node dissection (ILND) in melanoma patients. Ann Surg Oncol. 17, 2764-72

Chen Y et al. (2008) Reliability of Measurements For Lymphedema in Breast Cancer Patients. Am J Phys Med Rehabil. 87, 33-38

Cheville A et al. The Grading of Lymphedema in Oncology Clinical Trials. (2003) Seminars in Radiation Oncology. 13, 214-225

Cirelli, M. (1962). Treatment of inflammation and edema with bromelain. Delaware Med J, 34,159-167.

Connell, FC (2009) et al Analysis of the coding regions of VEGFR3 and VEGFC in Milroy disease and other primary lymphoedemas. Hum Genetics 124, 625-631

Cooper, R et al. (2009) Cutaneous Infections in Lymphoedema. Journal of Lymphoedema, 4, 44-48

Corica, GF et al (2006) Objective measurement of scarring by multiple assessors: is the tissue tonometer a reliable option? J Burn Care Res. 27, 520-523

Cormier, J et al (2010) Lymphedema beyond breast cancer: A systematic review and meta-analysis of cancer-related secondary lymphedema. Cancer 116 5138- 5149.

Cornu-Thenard, A et al. (2007) Superimposed Elastic Stockings: Pressure Measurements Dermatol Surg 33:269–275

Cotonat, A. (1989). Lymphangogue and pulsatile activities of Daflon 500 mg on canine thoracic lymph duct. International Angiology, 8, 15-18

Deltombe T et al. (2007) Reliability and limits of agreement of circumferential, water displacement and optoelectric volumetry in the measurement of upper limb lymphedema. Lymphology 40, 26-34

Didem, K et al (2005) The comparison of two different physiotherapy methods in treatment of lymphedema after breast surgery Breast Cancer Research and Treatment 93, 49–54

Dini, D. (1998). The role of peumatic compression in the treatment of postmastectomy lymphedema. A randomized phase III study. Ann Oncol. 9. 187- 190.

Executive Committee of International Society of Lymphology (2009) The Diagnosis and Treatment of Peripheral Lymphedema. Consensus Document of the International Society of Lymphology. Lymphology, 42, 51-60

Farrow, WP (2010) National Lymphedema Network: What is Lymphedema? http://www.lymphnet.org/lymphedemaFAQs/overview.htm

Farrow, WP (2010) Position Statement of the National Lymphedema Network –
Early Detection of LE. http://www.lymphnet.org/lymphedemaFAQs/positionPapers.htm

Farrow, WP (2010) Position Statement of the National Lymphedema Network –
Topic: The diagnosis and treatment of lymphedema

http://www.lymphnet.org/lymphedemaFAQs/positionPapers.htm
Fazhi Q et al, (2009)Treatment of upper limb lymphedema with combination of liposuction, myocutaneous flap transfer, and lymph-fascia grafting: A preliminary study. Microsurgery. 29, 29-34.
Ferrandez, J. (1996). Lymphoscintigraphic aspects of the effects of manual lymphatic drainage. J Mal Vasc, 21, 283-289
Ferrell RE (2008) Candidate Gene Analysis in Primary Lymphedema. Lymphat Res Biol 6, 69-76
Foldi E, et al. (2005).The Science of Lymphoedema Bandaging in Calne, S. Editor. European Wound
Management Association (EWMA). Focus Document: Lymphoedema Bandaging in Practice. London: MEP Ltd, 2-4
Franzcek U et al (1997) Combined physical therapy for lymphedema evaluated by fluorescence microlymphography and lymph capillary pressure measurements. J Vasc Res, 34, 306-311
Fu, M et al (2009) Breast Cancer Survivors' Experiences of Lymphedema-Related Symptoms J Pain Symptom Manage;38:849e859.
Fu, M.R et al. (2008). Breast Cancer-Related Lymphedema: Information, Symptoms, and Risk Reduction Behaviors. J Nurs Scholarsh, 40, 341-348.
Fu, M.R., Chen, C., Haber, J., Guth, A. & Axelrod, D. (2010). The Effects of Providing Information about Lymphedema on the Cognitive and Symptom Outcomes of Breast Cancer Survivors. Annals of Surgical Oncology, 17(7), 1847-53. Epub 2010 Feb 6.PMID: 20140528. DOI 10.1245/s10434-010-0941-3
Gaby, A. (1995). The story of bromelain. Nutr Healing, 3, 4-11.
Gergich, N et al (2008) Preoperative assessment enables the early diagnosis and successful treatment of lymphedema. Cancer. 112, 2809-2819.
Gloviczki, P. (1999). Principles of surgical treatment of chronic lymphoedema. International Angiology, 18 42-46.
Godoy J et al. (2007) Prevalence of cellulitis and erysipelas in post-mastectomy patients after breast cancer. Arch Med Sci, 3, 249-251
Gordon, K (2007). A guide to lymphedema. Expert Review of Dermatology, 2 (6) 741-752[115] Gultig, O (2005) Lymphoedema bandaging for the head, breast and genitalia. In Calne, S. Editor. European Wound Management Association (EWMA). Focus Document: Lymphoedema bandaging in practice. London: MEP Ltd, 2-4
Gur, A et al. (2009) Risk factors for breast cancer-related upper extremity lymphedema. Central European Journal of Medicine. 4, 65-70
Gupta, N et al. (2006) A female with hemihypertrophy and chylous ascites- Klippel Trenaunay Syndrome or Proteus Syndrome: a diagnostic dilemma. Clin Dysmorphol. 15: 229-231
Hafner, A et al. (2005) Combined modality treatment of lymphedema using the Reid Sleeve and the Biocompression Optiflow system. Journal of Clinical Oncology. 23(s), 592.
Hammer JB et al. (2007) Lymphedema Therapy Reduces the Volume of Edema and Pain in Patients with Breast Cancer. Annals of Surgical Oncology 14, 1904– 1908.
Hammond, T et al. (2009) Programmable Intermittent Pneumatic Compression as a Component of Therapy for Breast Cancer Treatment–Related Truncal and Arm

Lymphedema Home Health Care Management Practice Online First, doi:10.1177/1084822309343421

Hayes S et al. (2005) Comparison of Methods to Diagnose Lymphoedema among breast cancer survivors: 6 month follow up. Br Ca Res Treat. 89, 221-226

Hayes S et al. (2008) Lymphedema secondary to breast cancer: how choice of measure influences diagnosis, prevalence, and identifiable risk factors. Lymphology 41,18-28

Hayes, S et al.(2008) Lymphedema After Breast Cancer: Incidence, Risk Factors, and Effect on Upper Body Function. J Clin Oncol 28, 3536-3542

Helyer, L. K., Varnic, M., Le, L. W., Leong, W., & McCready, D. (2010). Obesity is a risk factor for developing postoperative lymphedema in breast cancer patients. The Breast Journal, 16(1), 48-54.

Hinrichs CS, et al. (2004) The effectiveness of complete decongestive physiotherapy for the treatment of lymphedema following groin dissection for melanoma. J Surg Oncol. 85: 187–192

Hormes, JM et al. (2010) Impact of lymphedema and arm symptoms on quality of life in breast cancer survivors. Lymphology 43, 1-13

Jahr, S et al. (2008) Effect of treatment with low intensity and extremely low frequency electrostatic fields (deep oscillation) on breast tissue and pain on patients with secondary breast lymphoedema. J Rehabil Med. 40, 645-650

Johansson K, et al. (2005) Low intensity resistance exercise for breast cancer patients with arm lymphedema with or without compression sleeve. Lymphology 38,167-80

Johnstone, PA et al. (2006) Role of patient adherence in maintenance of results after manipulative therapy for lymphedema J Soc Integr Oncol. 4, 125-9

Kelly, G. (1996). Bromelain: a literature review and discussion of its therapeutic applications. Altern Med Rev, 1, 243-257.

Kim, D.I. (2004). Excisional surgery for chronic advanced lymphedema. Surgery Today, 34, 134-137

Kim SJ et al. (2007) Effect of Complex Decongestive Therapy and the Quality of Life in Breast Cancer Patients with Unilateral Lymphedema. Lymphology 40, 143- 151.

King, T. (2001). Physical properties of short-stretch compression bandages used to treat lymphedema. Am J Occup Ther, 55, 573-576

Ko, D. (1998). Effective treatment of lymphedema of the extremities. Arch Surg, 133, 452-458

Koshima, I. (2000). Supermicrosurgical lymphaticovenular anastomosis for the treatment of lymphedema in the upper extremities. J Reconstr Microsurg, 16, 437-442.

Koul et al. (2007) Efficacy of complete decongestive therapy and manual lymphatic drainage on treatment related lymphedema in breast cancer. Int. J. Radiation Oncology Biol. Phys, 67, 841–846.

Krasin M, McCall A, King S, Olson M, Emami B. Evaluation of a standard breast tangent technique: a dose-volume analysis of tangential irradiation using three-dimensional tools. *Int J Radiat Oncol Biol Phys* 2000;47:327–333.

Lacomba, M (2010) Effectiveness of early physiotherapy to prevent lymphoedema after surgery for breast cancer: randomised, single blinded, clinical trial

Land S, Kopec J, Julian T, Brown A, Anderson S, Krag D, Christian N, Constantino J, Wolmark N, Ganz P. Patient-reported outcomes in sentinel node-negative adjuvant breast cancer patients receiving sentinel-node biopsy or axillary dissection:

National Surgical Adjuvant Breast and Bowel Project phase III protocol B-32. *J Clin Oncol.* 2010;28(25):3929-3936.

Lasinski, B. (2002). Comprehensive lymphedema management: results of a five- year follow-up. Lymphology, 35, 301-305.

Lawrence, S. (2008) Use of a Velcro Wrap System in the management of lower limb lymphoedema/oedema. Journal of Lymphoedema, 3, 65-70

Lawrence, S. (2008) Use of a Velcro Wrap System in the management of lower limb lymphoedema/oedema. Journal of Lymphoedema, 3, 65-70

Lerner R (2000) Effects of compression bandaging. Lymphology 33: 69

Lewin, J et al. (2010) Preliminary Experience With Head and Neck Lymphedema and Swallowing Function in Patients Treated for Head and Neck Cancer. Perspectives on Swallowing and Swallowing Disorders. Dysphagia 19, 45-52

Loprinzi, C. (1999). Lack of effect of coumarin in women with lymphedema after treatment for breast cancer. N Engl J Med. 340, 346-50.

Lund, E. (2000). Exploring the use of CircAid legging in the management of lymphoedema. Int J Palliat Nurs, 6, 383-391

Mallon, E. (1994). Lymphedema and wound healing. Clin Dermatol,12, 89-93

Mansel RE, Fallowfield L, Kissin M, Goyal A, Newcombe RG, Dixon JM, Yiangou C, Horgan K, Bundred N, Monypenny I, England D, Sibbering M, Abdullah TI, Barr L, Chetty U, Sinnett DH, Fleissig A, Clarke D, Ell PJ. Randomized multicenter trial of sentinel node biopsy versus standard axillary treatment in operable breast cancer: *The ALMANIC trial. J Natl Cancer Inst* 2006;98:599-609.

Maus, E. (2010) Near-infrared fluorescence imaging of lymphatics in head and neck lymphedema. Head and Neck. Online November 12, 2010. DOI: 10.1002/hed.21538

Mayrovitz, H (2009) Assessing lymphedema by tissue indentation force and local tissue water. Lymphology 42, 88-98

Mayrovitz, H (2009) Suitability of single tissue dielectric constant measurements to assess local tissue water in normal and lymphedematous skin. Clin Physiol Imaging 29: 123-127

Mayrovitz, HN. (2007) Interface pressures produced by two different types of lymphedema therapy devices. Phys Ther 87, 1379-1388

Mayrovitz HN (2009)The standard of care for lymphedema: current concepts and physiological considerations.Lymphat Res Biol 7,101-8

Mclaughlin S, Wright M, Morris K, Sampson M, Brockway J, Hurley K, Riedel E, Van ZeeK. Prevalence of lymphedema in women with breast cancer 5 years after sentinel lymph node biopsy or axillary dissection: Patient perceptions and precautionary behaviors. *J Clin Oncol.* 2008; 26:5220-5226.

Meek AG. Breast radiotherapy and lymphedema. Cancer. 1998;83:2788-2797

McNeely, M. (2004). The addition of manual lymph drainage to compression therapy for breast cancer related lymphedema: a randomized controlled trial Breast Cancer Res Treat, 86, 95-106.

Micke O, et al. (2003) Selenium in the treatment of radiation-associated secondary lymphedema. Int J Radiat Oncol Biol Phys . 56, 40-9

Miller, T.A. (1998). Staged skin and subcutaneous excision for lymphedema: a favorable report of long-term results. Plast Reconstr Surg, 102,1486-498.

Mirnajafi, A et al. (2004) A New Technique for Measuring Skin Changes of Patients with Chronic Postmastectomy Lymphedema. Lymph Res Biol. 2, 82-85

Miranda F et al. (2001) Effect of Sequential Intermittent Pneumatic Compression On Both Leg Lymphedema Volume and On Lymph Transport As SemiQuantitatively Evaluated by Lymphoscintigraphy. Lymphology 34 135-141.

Mondry T et al (2004) Prospective trial of complete decongestive therapy for upper extremity lymphedema after breast cancer therapy, 10, 42-8

Moseley A, et al. (2008) Exercise for Limb Lymphoedema: evidence that it is beneficial. J Lymphoedema. 3,51-56

Murphy, B et al. 2010, Late-effect laryngeal oedema/lymphoedema. Journal of Lymphoedema, 5, 92-93

Mustian, K et al. (2009). Exercise for the Management of Side Effects and Quality of Life among Cancer Survivors. Curr Sports Med Rep 8; 325-330

NLN Position Paper (2011) Risk Reduction Practices (2011) Retrieved 7-15-11, from http://www.lymphnet.org/pdfDocs/nlnriskreduction.pdf

Norman, S.A., Localio, A.R., Kallan, M.J. (2010). Risk Factors for Lymphedema after Breast Cancer Treatment. *Cancer Epidemiol Biomarkers, (19), 2737*

Olszewski, W (2009) Anatomical distribution of tissue fluid and lymph in soft tissues of lower limbs in obstructive lymphedema-hints for physiotherapy. Phlebolymphology. 16, 283-289.

Omar A et al. (2010) Treatment of Post Mastectomy Lymphedema with laser therapy: double blind placebo control randomized study. J Surg Research, 165, 82-90

Orecchia R, Huscher A, Leonardi MC, Gennari R, Galimberti C, Garibaldi C, Rondi E, Bianchi LC, Zurrida S, Franzetti S. Irradiation with standard tangential breast fields in patients treated with conservative surgery and sentinel node biopsy: using a three-dimensional tool to evaluate the first level coverage of the axillary nodes. *British Journal of Radiology 2005;78:51-54.*

Partsch, H. (1980). Experimental observations on the effect of a pressure wave massage apparatus (Lympha-Press) in lymphedema. Phlebologie Proktologie. 80. 124-128

Petrek, JA (2001) Lymphedema in a Cohort of Breast Carcinoma Survivors: 20 years after diagnosis. Cancer. 92, 1368-77

Piller et al. Placebo controlled trial of mild electrical stimulation. Journal of Lymphoedema, 2010, Vol 5, No 1. 15-25.

Piller, N, (2009) Phlebolymphoedema/chronic venous lymphatic insufficiency: an introduction to strategies for detection, differentiation and treatment. Phlebology 24:51-55

Rabinovitch R, Ballonoff A, Newman F, Finlayson C. Evaluation of breast sentinel lymph node coverage by standard radiation therapy fields. *Int J Radiat Oncol Biol Phys.* 2008;70(5):1468-1471.

Rasmussen J et al.(2009) Lymphatic Imaging in Humans with Near-Infrared Fluorescence. Curr Opin Biotechnol. 20-74-82

Rasmussen J et al (2010) Human Lymphatic Architecture and Dynamic Transport Imaged Using Near-infrared Fluorescence. Transl Oncol.; 3362–372

Ridner, S.(2009) The PsychoSocial Impact of Lymphedema. Lymphat Res Biol. 7, 109–112

Ridner S, et al. (2007) Comparison of upper limb volume measurement techniques and arm symptoms between healthy volunteers and individuals with known lymphedema Lymphology 40, 35-46

Ridner, S et al. (2008) Home-based lymphedema treatment in patients with cancer-related lymphedema or noncancer-related lymphedema. Oncol Nurs Forum. 35, 671-80

Ridner, S., Dietrich, M., Stewart, B., & Armer, J. (2011). Body mass index and breast cancer treatment-related lymphedema. Supportive Care in Cancer, 1-5.

Rockson, S et al. (2007) Bioimpedance analysis in the assessment of lymphoedema diagnosis and management. J Lymphoedema. 2, 44-48.

Salgado CJ, Sassu P, Gharb BB, et al. Radical reduction of upper extremity lymphedema with preservation of perforators. Ann Plast Surg. Sep 2009;63(2):302-6

Schlembach PJ, Buchholz TA, Ross MI, Kirsner SM, Salas GJ, Strom EA, McNeese MD, Perkins GH, Hunt KK. Relationship of sentinel and axillary level I-II lymph nodes to tangential fields used in breast irradiation. *Int J Radiat Oncol Biol Phys* 2001;51:671–678.

Schmitz, KH et al. (2009) Weight Lifting in Women with Breast-Cancer–Related Lymphedema N Engl J Med 361:664-73.

Schumacher, M, et al. (2008)Treatment of Venous Malformations-comparison to lymphatic malformations. Lymphology. 41, 139-146

Segers P, Belgrado JP, LeDuc A, et al. Excessive pressure in multichambered cuffs used for sequential compression therapy. Phys Ther. 2002; 82:1000-1008

Shaw, S et al. (2007) A Randomized Controlled Trial of Weight Reduction as a Treatment for Breast Cancer-related Lymphedema. Cancer, 110, 1868–74

Siebert U, et al. (2002) Efficacy, routine effectiveness, and safety of horsechestnut seed extract in the treatment of chronic venous insufficiency. A meta-analysis of randomized controlled trials and large observational studies. Int Angiol. 4, 305-315

Shih, Y. (2009) Incidence,Treatment Costs, and Complications of Lymphedema After Breast Cancer Among Women of Working Age: A 2-Year Follow-Up Study. JCO 27, 2007-2014

Slavin SA et al.(1999) Return of lymphatic function after flap transfer for acute lymphedema. Ann Surg. 229,421-7

Smith B et al. (2010) Lymphedema Management in Head and Neck Cancer. Current Opinions in Otolaryngology and Head and Neck Surgery. 18,153-158

Smitt M, Goffinet D. Utility of three-dimensional planning for axillary node coverage with breast-conserving radiation therapy: early experience. *Radiology* 1999;210:221–226.

Soran, A et al. (2006) Breast Cancer Related Lymphedema-What are the Significant Predictors and how they affect the severity of lymphedema. Breast J, 12, 536-43

Szolnoky et al.(2009) Intermittent Pneumatic Compression Acts Synergistically With Manual Lymphatic Drainage In Complex Decongestive Therapy. Lymphology 42,188-194

Szuba, A et al (2000) Decongestive lymphatic therapy for patients with cancer- related or primary lymphedema. Am J Med. 109, 296-300

Szuba, A et al (2003) Diagnosis and treatment of concomitant venous obstruction in patients with secondary lymphedema. J Vasc Intervent Radiol. 13,799-803

Szuba, A et al. (2003) The third circulation: radionuclide lymphoscintigraphy in the evaluation of lymphedema. J Nucl Med, 44, 43-57

Szuba (2007) Presence of Axillary lymph nodes and lymph drainage within arms of women with and without breast cancer-related lymphedema. Lymphology 40- 81-86

Takeda A, Shigematsu N, Kondo M, Amemiya A, Kawaguchi O, Sato M, Kutsuki S, Toya K, Ishibashi R, Kawase T, Tsukamoto N, Kubo A. The modified tangential irradiation technique for breast cancer: how to cover the entire axillary region. *Int J Radiat Oncol Biol Phys* 2000;46:815–822.

Takeda A, Shigematsu N, Ikeda T, Kawaguchi O, Kutsuki S, Ishibashi R, Kunieda E, Takemasa K, Ito H, Uno T, Jinno H, Kubo A. Evaluation of novel modified tangential irradiation technique for breast cancer patients using dose-volume histograms. *Int J Radiat Oncol Biol Phys*2004;58(4):1280-1288.

Taylor, H. (1993). A double blind clinical trial of hydroxyethylrutosides in obstructive arm lymphodema. Phlebology, 8, 22-28.

Tidhar, D et al. (2010) Aqualymphatic therapy in women who suffer from breast cancer treatment-related lymphedema: a randomized controlled study. Support Care Cancer. 18: 383-392

Thomas, RC et al. (2007) Reduction of lymphedema using complete decongestive therapy: roles of prior radiation therapy and extent of axillary dissection. J Soc Integrat Oncol.5, 87-91

Unno, N et al. (2008) Quantitative Lymph Imaging for Assessment of Lymph Function using Indocyanine Green Fluorescence Lymphography. Eur J Vasc Endovasc Surg 36, 230-236

Unno N et al. (2010) A novel method of measuring human lymphatic pumping using indocyanine green fluorescence lymphography. J Vasc Surg 52, 946-52

Vaillant, L. (2002). Infectious complications of lymphedema. Rev Med Interne, 23, 403-407

Veronesi U, Paganelli G, Galimberti V, Viale G, Zurrida S, Bedoni M, Costa A, de Cicco C, Geraghty JG, Luini A, Sacchini V, Veronesi P. Sentinel-node biopsy to avoid axillary dissection in breast cancer with clinically negative lymph-nodes. *Lancet.* 1997; 349(9069): 1864-1867.

Veronesi U, Paganelli G, Viale G, Luini A, Zurrida S, Galimberti V, Intra M, Veronesi P, Robertson C, Maisonneuve P, Renne G, De Cicco, C, De Licoa F, Genari R. A randomized comparison of sentinel-node biopsy with routine axillary dissection in breast cancer. *N Engl J Med.* 2003;349:546-53

Vignes, S. (2002). Role of surgery in the treatment of lymphedema. Rev. Med Interne. 23, 426-430.

Vignes, S (2006) Recurrence of lymphoedema-associated cellulitis (erysipelas) under prophylactic antibiotherapy: a retrospective cohort study JEADV,20:, 818– 822

Wang, Z. (2005) Clinical Report of congenital lymphatic malformations and partial gigantism of the hands associated with a heterogenous karyotype. Am J Medical Genetics 132A, 106-107

Ward, L, (2006) Bioelectrical Impedance Analysis: Proven Utility in Lymphedema Risk Assessment and Therapeutic Monitoring. Lymph Res Biol. 4, 51-56

Warren, A et al. (2007) Lymphedema: A comprehensive review. Annals of Plastic Surgery, 59, 464-472

Weiss, J. (2002). The effect of complete decongestive therapy on the quality of life of patients with peripheral lymphedema. Lymphology, 35, 46-58.

Weiss M, et al (2003) Dynamic lymph flow imaging in patients with oedema of the lower limb for evaluation of the functional outcome after autologous lymph vessel transplantation: an 8-year follow-up study. Eur J Nucl Med Mol Imaging; 30, 202-206.

Wernicke AG, Goodman RL, Turner BC, Komarnicky LT, Curran WJ, Christos PJ, Khan I, Vandris K, Parashar B, Nori D, Chao KS. A 10 year follow up of treatment outcomes in patients with early stage breast cancer and clinically negative axillary nodes treated with tangential breast irradiation following sentinel lymph node dissection or axillary clearance. *Breast Cancer Res Treat.* 2010;125(3):893-902.

Wernicke AG, Shamis M, Sidhu KK, et al. Complication rate in patients with negative axillary nodes 10-years after local breast radiotherapy following sentinel lymph node dissection or axillary clearance. *Am J Clin Oncol* 2011 (in press).

Williams, A (2005) Practical Guidance on Lymphoedema Bandaging of the Upper and Lower Extremities. In Calne, S. Editor. European Wound Management Association (EWMA). Focus Document: Lymphoedema bandaging in practice. London: MEP Ltd, 10-14

Williams, AF et al (2002) A randomized controlled crossover study of manual lymphatic drainage therapy in women with breast cancer-related lymphoedema. European Journal of Cancer Care 11, 254–261

Wong JS, Taghian AG, Bellon JR, Keshaviah A, Smith BL, Winer EP, Silver B, Harris JR. Tangential radiotherapy without axillary surgery in early-stage breast cancer: results of a prospective trial. *Int J Radiat Oncol Biol Phys.* 2008;72(3):866-870.

Yamamoto et al. (2008) Study of Edema Reduction Patterns During the Treatment Phase of Complex Decongestive Physiotherapy for Extremity Lymphedema. Lymphology 41 80-86

Yamazaki, A. (1988). Clinical experience using pneumatic massage therapy for edematous limbs over the last 10 years. Angilogy. 39. 154-163.

Yasuhara, H. (1996). A study of the advantages of elastic stockings for leg lymphedema. Int Angiol, 15, 272-277

4

Preparing for and Coping with Breast Cancer-Related Lymphedema

M. Elise Radina[1] and Mei R. Fu[2]
[1]*Miami University*
[2]*New York University*
USA

1. Introduction

Despite recent trends indicating that new diagnoses of breast cancer have decreased slightly, the American Cancer Society estimates that there will be 207,090 new cases of invasive breast cancer and 54,010 new cases of in situ (i.e., early stage) breast cancer that are likely to have developed in 2010 (American Cancer Society, 2010). Given that the 5-year survival rate for breast cancer is now 90% and that the National Cancer Institute estimates that there were approximately 2.5 million women living in 2006 who had a history of breast cancer (American Cancer Society, 2010; Horner et al., 2009), experiencing breast cancer is increasingly about survivorship. Breast cancer survivors are at lifetime risk for developing lymphedema, a chronic condition that occurs in up to 40% of this population (Armer, Stewart, & Shook, 2009; American Cancer Society, 2007; Ferlay, Bray, Pisani, & Parkin, 2004). Lymphedema involves the accumulation of protein-rich fluid that impacts physical, functional, and psychosocial health and well-being. Second only to breast cancer recurrence, lymphedema is the most dreaded outcome of breast cancer treatment. Research has shown that women with breast cancer-related lymphedema report their most frequent action for management of lymphedema symptoms is no action (Armer & Whitman, 2002). This indicates that patient education about self-care is critical for effective self-management and risk reduction. Given the distressing and chronic nature of breast cancer-related lymphedema, there are both individual and family level psychosocial impacts related to the onset and long-term management.

This chapter is aimed at addressing real and present concerns for both patients and their family members regarding breast cancer-related lymphedema. All too often these individuals are poorly prepared to cope with the potential or actual realities of living with this physically limiting chronic condition. At the same time, many patients and family members report being both unaware that lymphedema was a possible outcome of breast cancer treatment and that medical staff, in particular oncologist and surgeons, are not well informed and/or not helpful in guiding them on how to cope. What is offered in this chapter is an overview of the condition with special attention paid to informing readers (e.g., physicians, nursing, social workers, family therapists, and others who work with patients and their families) so that they might be better equipped to serve patients and the family members. Thus, the focus of this chapter is thus two-fold: 1) patient (and family member/ caregiver) education regarding strategies for early detection, risk reduction, and management/self-care and 2) individual and family level psychosocial impacts of coping with breast cancer-related lymphedema.

2. Defining breast cancer-related lymphedema

Breast cancer-related lymphedema, a syndrome of abnormal swelling and multiple distressing symptoms, is a major adverse effect of breast cancer treatment (Fu & Rosedale, 2009). Lymphedema is a chronic condition involving accumulation of protein-rich fluid that impacts physical, functional, and psychosocial health and well-being (Beaulac, McNair, Scott, LaMorte, & Kavanah, 2002; Geller, Vacek, O'Brien, & Secker-Walker, 2003; Hull, 1998; Radina & Armer, 2004; Voogd et al., 2003). (Figure 1).

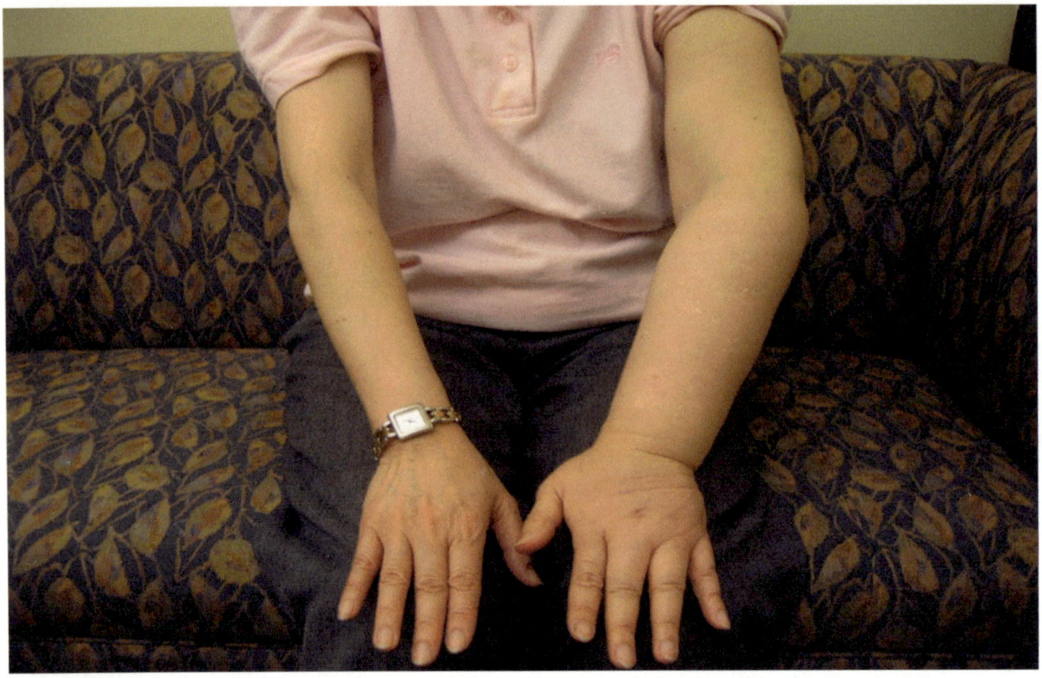

Fig. 1. Example of Breast Cancer-related Lymphedema.

While the exact cause of breast cancer-related lymphedema is unknown, evidence suggests that some cancer treatments may increase the risk of developing breast cancer-related lymphedema; risks that include the surgical removal of lymphatic vessels and nodes and the development of tissue fibrosis that sometimes follow radiation treatments, infection, or surgery (Kwan et al., 2002). Common breast cancer treatments damage and potentially weaken the lymph nodes and the vessels carrying lymph fluid, which may then compromise the effectiveness of the valves in the lymph vessels (Smith, 1998). The result is the accumulation of lymph fluid in the tissues of the arm, hand, chest, back, and neck (Berne & Levy, 1996). Changes in physical appearance and limitations created by lymphedema can affect physical and psychological health as well as interpersonal relationships (Casley-Smith, 1992; Passik & McDonald, 1998; Passik, Newman, Brennan, & Tunkel, 1995; Radina, Watson, & Faubert, 2009; Thomas-MacLean, Miedema, & Tatemichi, 2005). Although women with breast cancer-related lymphedema report a variety of physical symptoms (e.g., pain, heaviness, tenderness, numbness, limited range of motion, and stiffness), arm swelling is the most common (Armer, Radina, Porock, & Culbertson, 2003; Coster, Polle, & Fallowfield, 2001; Thomas-MacLean et al., 2005). In addition, those coping with this chronic, sometimes disabling, condition are subject to frustrating physical limitations (e.g., being unable to lift heavy objects; reducing activities that require repetitive motions with the arm; keeping the arm elevated) (Radina & Armer, 2001; Ridner, 2002).

3. Diagnosis of breast cancer-related lymphedema

Early diagnosis of breast cancer-related lymphedema remains a clinical challenge. Traditionally, lymphedema has been clinically diagnosed by healthcare professionals' observations of swelling, and has often arbitrarily been defined in research as a 2-cm increase in limb girth, a 200-mL or more increase in limb volume, or a 5% or greater limb volume change (Armer et al., 2004; Cormier et al., 2009; Stout et al., 2008). Inconsistency in the criteria defining lymphedema and the use of different measures has posed tremendous difficulty in accurately diagnosing lymphedema (Armer & Stewart, 2005). Additional contributing factors to the challenge include failure to precisely evaluate symptoms related to lymphedema, co-existing conditions, insufficient knowledge and lack of awareness among healthcare professionals. Several diagnostic approaches have been used for diagnosing breast cancer-related lymphedema, including the patient's health history and physical examination, measures of limb volume, and lymph vessle imaging.

3.1 Health history and physical examination

Early and accurate diagnosis of breast cancer-related lymphedema is essential to prevent complications and achieve optimal management. A careful review of the patient's health history can promote accurate diagnosis to rule out other medical conditions that may cause similar symptoms. Such medical conditions include recurrent cancer, deep vein thrombosis, chronic venous insufficiency, diabetes, hypertension, cardiac and renal disease. These alternative diagnoses should be ruled out before establishing a diagnosis of lymphedema and referring the patient for lymphedema therapy.

A four-stage system (Table 1) can be used to facilitate physical examination to classify lymphedema in terms of skin condition and swelling (International Society of Lymphedema ([ISL], 2003). Within each stage, severity of lymphedema based on volume difference can be assessed as mild (<20% increase), moderate (20-40% increase), or severe (>40% increase). It should be noted that a clinical diagnosis of lymphedema in the current practice patterns is very often made when swelling becomes visually evident and is usually classified as "mild" lymphedema. Mild lymphedema is often defined as an initially reversible. However, by the time lymphedema is visually observable (as described in the Stage 2) it has already evolved into the irreversible advanced stages.

Stages	Presentations
0 Latent or sub-clinical condition	• No noticeable swelling • No pitting • A feeling of heaviness • Existing months or years before overt swelling occurs
i. Early accumulation of lymph fluid	• Pitting swelling • Visible swelling
ii. Increased or chronic swelling	• Pitting swelling • Hardened and thickened tissue
iii. Lymphostatic elephantiasis	• Absence of pitting swelling • Enlarged and obvious swelling of the affected limb • Hardness, thickness, and toughness of skin • Lymph leaking through damaged skin

Table 1. Staging of Lymphedema (International Society of Lymphedema ([ISL], 2003)

Symptom assessment is essential since very often observable swelling and measurable volume changes are absent during the initial development of lymphedema, but patients may report such symptoms as heaviness, tightness, firmness, pain, or numbness (Cormier et al., 2009; Fu & Rosedale, 2009). These symptoms may be the earliest indicator of increasing interstitial pressure changes associated with lymphedema (Kosir et al., 2001). As the fluid increases, the limb may become visibly swollen with an observable increase in limb size. Recent research shows that limb volume change (LVC) by the infra-red perometer has significantly increased as breast cancer survivors' reports of swelling, heaviness, tenderness, firmness, tightness, and aching have increased (Cormier et al., 2009). On average, breast cancer survivors reported 4.2 symptoms for survivors with $<5.0\%$ LVC; 5.5 symptoms for 5.0-9.9% LVC, 7.0 symptoms for 10.0-14.9% LVC, and 12.5 symptoms for $> 15\%$ LVC, respectively ($p<0.001$) (Cormier et al., 2009). Because early intervention is believed to yield better patient outcomes, the presence of lymphedema symptoms should warrant institution of early interventions (Armer, Radina, Porock, & Culbertson, 2003; Armer et al., 2004; Foeldi et al., 2003). In addition, experience of symptoms has elicited tremendous distress in breast cancer survivors and exerted negative impact on their quality of lives (Fu & Rosedale 2009; Pyszel et al., 2006). Symptoms should be one of the major patient-centered clinical outcomes for evaluating the effectiveness of lymphedema treatment (Armer et al., 2005; Sitzia, Stanton, & Badger, 1997). A symptom checklist (Table 2) may be used for symptom assessment.

The following questions are about symptoms in your affected arm, hand, breast, axilla (under arm), or chest today or in the past three months.					
	How Severe?				
Have you had ___?	No 0	A little 1	Somewhat 2	Quite a bit 3	Very Severe 4
1. Shoulder					
2. Elbow					
3. Wrist					
4. Fingers					
5. Arm					
6. Hand or arm swelling					
7. Breast swelling					
8. Chest wall swelling					
9. Firmness					
10. Tightness					
11. Heaviness					
12. Toughness or thickness of skin					
13. Stiffness					
14. Tenderness					
15. Hotness/increased temperature					
16. Redness					
17. Blistering					
18. Pain/aching/soreness					
19. Numbness					
20. Burning					
21. Stabbing					
22. Tingling (pins and needles)					
23. Arm or hand fatigue					
24. Arm or hand weakness					

Table 2. Example of Symptom Checklist - Breast Cancer & Lymphedema Symptom Experience Index

Physical examination and symptom assessment can also help to differentiate if the onset of lymphedema following breast cancer treatment is gradual or sudden (Fu et al., 2009). It is still not fully understood why some patients are more prone to fluid build-up than others even with similarity in surgical treatment, numbers of lymph nodes removed, chemotherapy and radiotherapy. With gradual onset, noticeable swelling is often absent initially, but patients may report feelings of tightness and heaviness in the previous year, visible and measurable lymphedema typically occurs two to five years after treatment, but it can also happen as many as 15 to 30 years later (Armer et al., 2003; Petrek, Senie, Peters, & Rosen, 2001). With sudden onset, swelling develops rapidly, usually within 24 hours and often breast cancer survivors are able to identify the triggers, such as air travel, infection, or injuries (e.g., cuts, insect bites, pinpricks, burns) (Fu & Rosedale, 2009; Johansson, et al., 2002; Petrek et al., 2001). With infection (especially cellulitis) or injuries, breast cancer survivors usually experience sudden swelling with redness, elevated white blood cells, or elevated temperature (Foeldi et al., 2003). Very often, immediate administration of oral or IV antibiotics can clear the infection, while elevation of the limb helps to reduce the swelling. It is possible that early stage lymphedema (Stage 1 and 2) may continue to exist in a latent or sub-clinical state even when successfully treated at initial onset, sometimes presenting at later stages ten or more years after initial diagnosis of sudden onset of lymphedema (Brennan & Miller, 1998).

3.2 Measures of limb volume (LV)

Measuring LV is an objective way to quantifying lymphedema. However, quantifying lymphedema is a challenge because various measurement approaches have been used to define lymphedema and certain types of breast cancer-related lymphedema such as breast, shoulder, and truncal lymphedema cannot be quantified with current measurement technology. Methods of measuring limb volume LV include sequential circumference limb measurement, water displacement, infra-red perometry, and bioimpedance spectroscopy (Armer & Stewart, 2005; Petlund, 1991; Tierney, Aslam, Rennie, & Grace, 1996; Cornish, et al., 2001).

3.2.1 Sequential circumferential arm measurements

Measuring circumference is the most widely used diagnostic method. A flexible non-stretch tape measure for circumferences is usually used to assure consistent tension over soft tissue, muscle, and bony prominences (Armer et al., 2004; Petlund, 1991). Measurements are done on both affected and non-affected limbs at the hand proximal to the metacarpals, wrist, and then every 4 cm from the wrist to axilla or at minimum, six measurements are recommended: circumference at the mid-hand, wrist, elbow, upper arm just below the axilla, and at 10cm distal to and proximal to the lateral epicondyle on both arms (Armer et al., 2004; Callaway et al., 1988) The most common criterion for diagnosis has been a finding of ≥ 2 cm or >200 ml difference in limb volume as compared to the non-affected limb or 10% volume differences in the affected limb (Armer et al., 2004; Armer & Stewart, 2005; Mayrovitz, Simms, & MacDonald, 2000; Stanton et al., 2009).

Circumferential limb measurement has limited inter- and intra-rater reliability and costly in terms of training time and clinician's time for measurement (Armer & Stewart, 2005; Gerber, 1998). (Figure 2).

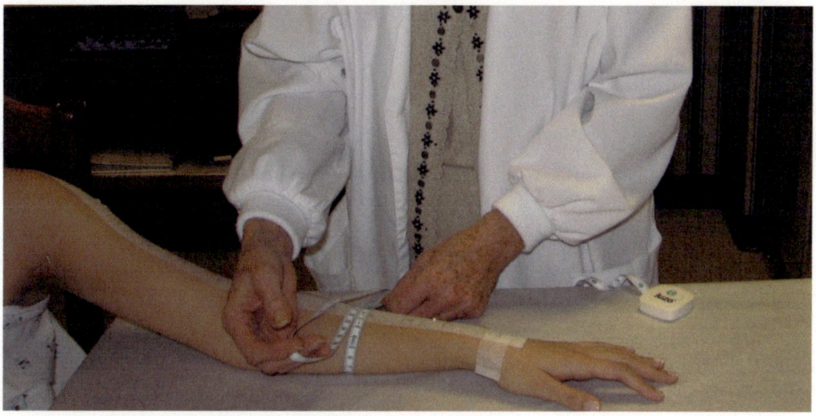

Fig. 2. Sequential Circumferential Arm Measurements

3.2.2 Water displacement

Water displacement is seldom used in clinical settings because of cumbersome spillover and hygienic concerns (Armer & Stewart, 2005; Gerber, 1998). Patients submerge the affected arm in a container filled with water and the overflow of water is caught in another container and weighed (Figure 3). This method does not provide data about localization of swelling or shape of the extremity (Petlund, 1991; Tierney et al., 1996). The method is contraindicated in patients with open skin lesions. Patients may find it difficult to hold the position for the time needed for the tank overflow to drain.

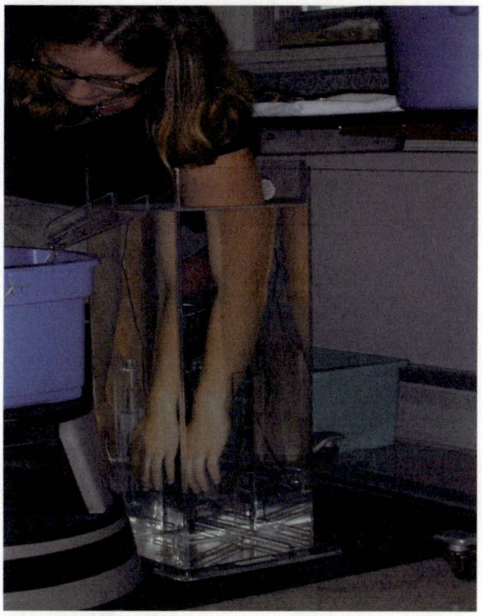

Fig. 3. Water Displacement

3.2.3 Infra-red perometry

The advent of infra-red perometry (also called optoelectronic volumetry), such as the perometer 350S (Juzo, Cuyahoga Falls, OH), enables reliable and accurate detection of 3% limb volume change (LVC) (Cormier et al., 2009; Stout et al., 2008). The perometer works in much the same manner as computed tomography but uses infrared light instead of X-rays (Petlund, 1991). There is no toxic effect to the patient. Perometry is performed on each arm as it is held horizontally with the patient standing comfortably (Figure 4). The perometer maps a 3-dimensional graph of the affected and non-affected extremities using numerous rectilinear light beams, and interfaces with a computer for data analysis and storage. A 3-dimensional limb image is generated and LV is calculated. This optoelectronic method has a standard deviation of 8.9 ml (arm), less than 0.5% of LV with repeated measuring (Armer & Stewart, 2005; Cormier et al., 2009). Because the perometer is capable of measuring bilateral lymphedema and localization of swelling as well as detecting a 3% LVC that enables detectable differences in quality of life (QOL) and symptom reporting, the optimal measure for lymphedema is the evaluation of LVC by the perometer (Armer & Stewart, 2005; Cormier et al., 2009; Stout et al., 2008).

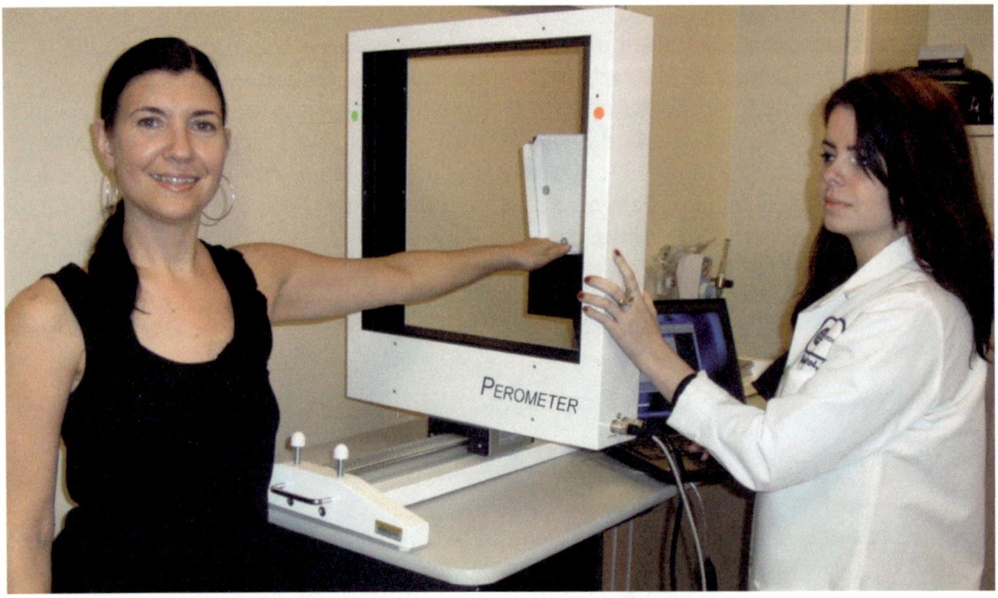

Fig. 4. Infra-red Perometry

3.2.4 Bioimpedance spectroscopy (BIS)

Bioelectrical impedance has been used to detect onset lymphedema and monitor results of lymphatic massage in clinical settings (Cornish, et al., 2001; Ridner, Montgomery, Hepworth, Stewart, & Armer, 2007; Ward, Bunce, Cornish, Mirolo, Thomas, & Jones, 1992; Ward, Essex, & Cornish, 2006). The Imp XCA® (Impedimed, Brisbane, Australia) uses a single frequency below 30 kHz to measure impedance and resistance of the extracellular fluid. The device uses the impedance ratio values between the unaffected and affected limb to determine arm lymphedema. Ratio means of 1.139 for at-risk dominant arms and 1.066 for at-risk non-dominant arms are indicators of arm lymphedema. The Imp XCA® uses the impedance ratio values to calculate a *Lymphedema Index [L-Dex]*. The L-Dex scale ranges from -10 to +10, which is equivalent to the impedance ratio from 0.935 to 1.139 for at-risk dominant arms and 0.862 to 1.066 for at-risk non-dominant arms, respectively. Each one standard unit in L-Dex is equivalent to the impedance ratio of 0.03. A patient is determined to have arm lymphedema or arm swelling if the patient's L-Dex exceeds the normal value of +10, i.e. exceed impedance ratio means of 1.139 for at-risk dominant arms and 1.066 for at-risk non-dominant arms, respectively (44). Measurement of arms takes less than five minutes when using the Imp-XCA® and results are immediately available to clinicians. However, the Imp XCA® is only capable of assessing unilateral lymphedema, unable to provide data about localization of swelling or shape of the extremity, and cannot be applied to patients with renal or heart failure, cardiac pacemaker or defibrillator, inability to lying down on the exam table, artificial limbs, or pregnancy as accurate measurement of lymphedema may not be possible. Continuous cost for electrodes is needed. (Figure 4).

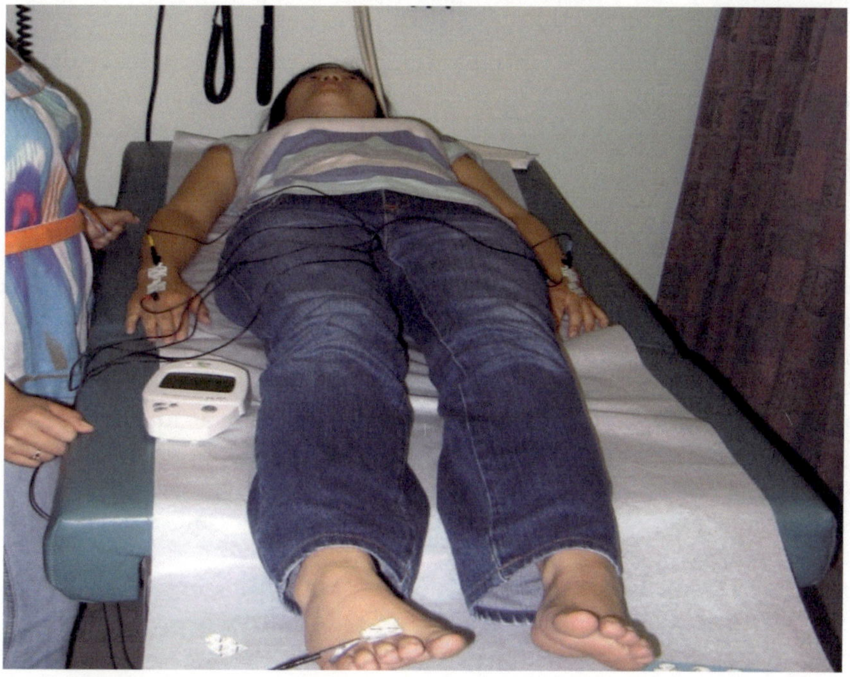

Fig. 5. Bioimpedance Spectroscopy (BIS).

3.3 Lymph vessel imaging

Lymphoscintigraphy (isotope lymphography) can ensure definite lymphedema diagnosis (Mortimer, 2003; Cambria et al., 1993). Lymphoscintigraphy employs a nuclear medicine to visualize the lymph vessel. With the patient supine, a radiolabelled macromolecular tracer (Tc-99m filtered [0.22 milli micron] or unfiltered sulfur colloid) is injected intradermally within one of the interdigital spaces of the affected limb using a 25-gauge needle in a 1 ml syringe (Cambria et al., 1993; Partsch, 1995; Ter et al., 1993). The injection is given between the index and middle finger in the web space for the upper limbs. Both sides are done simultaneously so that the affected limb can be compared to the unaffected limb. The lymphatic transport of the macromolecule is tracked with a gamma camera, and the rate of tracer disappearance from the injection site and the accumulation of counts within the lymph node are both quantified. Typical abnormalities observed in lymphedema include dermal backflow, absent or delayed transport of tracer, cross-over filling with retrograde backflow, and either absent or delayed visualization of the lymph nodes (Cambria et al., 1993; Partsch, 1995; Ter et al., 1993). However, lymphography is now rarely used in patients because of its potential to cause lymphatic injury and its inability to clarify function (Meek, 1998; Mortimer, 2003).

4. Treatment of breast cancer-related lymphedema

Treatment of lymphedema has been and continues to be a major healthcare challenge since no treatment can cure this chronic condition. Lymphedema treatment refers to therapies applied to help to slow the disease progression by reducing or maintaining swelling and relieving symptoms. Lymphedema therapy includes complete decongestive physiotherapy, pneumatic compression therapy (PCT), therapeutic exercises, surgery, and pharmacological therapy (Fu, 2005; Geller, Vacek, O'Brien, & Secker-Walker, 2003; ISL, 2003; Megens & Harris, 1998).

4.1 Complete decongestive therapy (CDT)

Complete decongestive therapy (also known as *complex decompressive physiotherapy, comprehensive decongestive treatment,* and *multimodal physical therapy*) is the standard of care for breast cancer-related lymphedema. CDT includes an initial reductive treatment phase followed by an ongoing maintenance phase. The reductive treatment phase involves 2-5 sessions per week for 3 to 8 weeks in a specialized lymphedema clinic until the reduction of fluid volume has reached a plateau. The reductive treatment phase of CDT consists of multiple components, including manual lymph drainage (MLD), multilayer, short-stretch compression bandaging, therapeutic exercise, skin care, education in self-management, and elastic compression garments (Davis, 1998; Megens & Harris, 1998). The reductive treatment phase should be reinstituted whenever swelling is exacerbated or whenever symptoms are worsened. Once the reductive treatment phase is completed, the maintenance phase starts in which the patient continues self-management with skin care and exercise, self MLD, and use of a compressive sleeve and gauntlet during the day and arm bandaging at night (Davis, 1998; Megens & Harris, 1998). The maintenance phase of CDT requires a lifelong self-management program with self MLD, exercise, skin care, and compression garments or bandages. Long-term volume reduction is as high as 50-63% in up to 79% of patients who are 100% compliant (Boris et al., 1997; Erickson et al., 2001; Foeldi et al., 2003; Rinerhart-Ayres, 1998). Yet, compliance with the prescribed self-management regimen during the maintenance phase is difficult for breast cancer survivors (Brennan & Miller, 1998; Fu, 2010). From the patient's perspective, the treatment for lymphedema itself is a constant reminder that prevents survivors from living a normal life (Fu, 2005; Fu & Rosedale, 2009).

4.2 Pneumatic compression therapy

Pneumatic compression therapy, also known as compression pump therapy, can be used daily for 30-60 minutes during the maintenance phase of CDT. Acceptable pneumatic compression device (PCD) should have multiple chambers delivering a sequential pressure. Caution must be used, however, because compression pumps can damage the vasculature. Furthermore, compression devices are contraindicated in patients with congestive heart failure, active infection, or deep venous thrombosis (Rockson et al., 1998). The recently developed PCD such as the Flexitouch® system is believed to be safer than the older PCD (Ridner et al., 2010). The Flexitouch® system is an advanced, programmable PCD that is cleared by the Food and Drug Administration for home use. This device is the only PCD designed to emulate the therapeutic techniques of MLD. Published studies and case reports suggest that breast cancer-related limb and truncal lymphedema may be effectively treated with the Flexitouch® system since the device includes garments to treat truncal swelling (Ridner et al., 2010).

4.3 Therapeutic exercises

Therapeutic exercises are individualized remedial exercises that consist of cardiovascular exercises, stretching, aerobic activity, and strength training. Therapeutic exercise is believed to increase lymph flow and protein absorption through repeated contraction and relaxation of muscles. Therapeutic exercise should be initiated by well-trained lymphedema therapists and then continued at home. One randomized controlled trial found that a 6-month intervention did not increase risk or add to symptoms of lymphedema (Ahmed et al., 2006). Other data also indicate that exercise as an individual therapy is neither a contraindication after breast cancer treatment nor does it decrease the risk of developing lymphedema (Ahmed et al., 2006; Schmitz et al., 2009; Johansson et al., 2005). For survivors with lymphedema, compression garments or compression bandages must be worn during exercise to counterbalance the buildup of interstitial fluid (Schmitz et al., 2009; Johansson et al., 2005).

4.4 Surgery

Surgical approaches are performed to debulk tissue or to divert lymphatic drainage (Casley-Smith, 1992; Cormier et al., 2011). Surgical treatment for breast cancer-related lymphedema is rarely performed except in severe and refractory cases to reduce the weight of the lymphedematous region, minimize the frequency of infectious and inflammatory episodes, and improve cosmesis and function. Surgical treatment includes: (1) excisional operations (e.g., debulking, amputation, and liposuction), (2) lymphatic reconstruction, and (3) tissue transfer procedures (e.g., lymph node transplantation, pedicled omentum, bone marrow stromal cell transplantation) (Cormier et al., 2011). For severe lymphedema, excisional operations and debulking procedures have been reported as effective methods to alleviate symptoms by removing fibrosclerotic connective tissue, excess adipose tissue, and excess skin. Various microsurgical techniques for lymphatic reconstruction have been attempted since the early 1960s, including the creation of anastomoses between lymphatic channels and adjacent veins, between lymph nodes and veins, and between distal and proximal lymphatics (Campisi et al., 2001; O'Brien et al., 1990). Lympho-lymphatic anastomosis and lymphatic grafting have been used as reconstructive techniques that are associated with improved patency over time (Brennan & Miller, 1998). A recent systematic review on surgical treatment for lymphedema revealed that the largest reported reductions were noted after excisional procedures (91.1%), lymphatic reconstruction (54.9%), and tissue transfer procedures (47.6%) (Cormier et al., 2011). Potential complications may occur with surgical management of lymphedema, such as recurrence of swelling, poor wound healing, and infection; thus surgical treatment should be considered only when other treatments fail, and with careful consideration of the benefits-to-risks ratio (Casley-Smith, 1992). It should be noted although these surgical approaches have shown promising results, nearly all the surgical procedures do not obviate the need for continued use of conventional therapies, including compression, for long-term maintenance (Cormier et al., 2011).

4.5 Pharmacological therapy

Pharmacological interventions to treat lymphedema include antibiotics for treatment of infections, benzopyrones, flavonoids, diuretics, hyaluronidase, pantothenic acid, and selenium (Bruns et al., 2003; Rockson et al., 1998; Olszewski et al., 2000). Although not approved by the US Food and Drug Administration (FDA), *benzopyrones* have drawn most of the attention as a pharmacologic approach to treat lymphedema (Rockson et al., 1998). Benzopyrones are believed to encourage protein breakdown and lead to a subsequent decrease in lymph fluid. One randomized controlled trial of benzopyrones and placebo showed a significant decrease in arm swelling after treatment for several months (Davis, 1998). Loprinzi (1999) conducted a controlled study on the effectiveness of coumarin compared with a placebo, and they concluded that coumarin was not effective for managing breast cancer-related lymphedema due to a high risk of hepatotoxicity. A Cochrane review found that it was not possible to draw conclusions about the effectiveness of benzopyrones in reducing and controlling lymphedema due to the poor quality of existing trials (Badger et al., 2004). Flavonoids, hyaluronidase, pantothenic acid, and selenium have also demonstrated limited efficacy (Olszewski et al., 2000; Bruns et al., 2003). Diuretics are not suitable for breast cancer-related lymphedema, as such medications only serve to increase protein concentrations in the interstitium and encourage increase in swelling, inflammation and fibrosis (Davis, 1998; Thiadens, 1998).

5. Risk reduction for and early detection of breast cancer-related lymphedema

5.1 Risk reduction

Breast cancer-related lymphedema is often under-diagnosed and undertreated. The complexity and variability of individual lymphatic system and the unpredictability of risk factors makes it difficult to predict which patients will ultimately develop lymphedema. For decades, to reduce the risk of lymphedema after breast cancer treatment, the focus has been on improving surgical treatment. Such improvements, including sentinel lymph node biopsy (SLNB) in which one to three sentinel lymph nodes are removed, and breast-conserving surgery (BCS) in which only the cancerous part of the breast is removed (Armer et al., 2004), have saved patients with node-negative disease from unnecessary axillary lymph node dissection (ALND) and mastectomy (Boneti et al., 2008; Giuliano et al, 2011).

While lymphedema and symptoms have been reported less frequently in women who underwent SLNB only, lymphedema has by no means becomes a minor or disappearing problem. Data from recent studies have revealed that lymphedema remains a significant complication of breast cancer treatment, occurring in 20% to 47% of cases after ALND and in 3% to 17% after SLNB (Cormier et al., 2009; Paskett et al., 2007; Langer et al., 2007; McLaughlin et al., 2008). It is very important to note that surgical removal of lymph nodes remains the optimal choice for treating breast cancer with positive cancerous lymph nodes (Boneti et al., 2008; Giuliano et al, 2011, Langer et al., 2007). Each year in the US, more than 190,000 women are diagnosed with invasive breast cancer and many of them undergo removal of positive lymph nodes despite the use of SLNB, predisposing the women to a life-time risk for lymphedema.

In addition, radiation exposure is associated with trauma to the lymphatic system, and current standard of care includes BCS and SLNB together with radiation therapy to breast and /or axilla. Recent innovative approaches to radiotherapy include the single-day targeted intraoperative radiotherapy delivered by the Targit machine (Enderling, Anderson, Chaplain, Munro, & Vaidya, 2006; Vaidya et al., 2006) and the 5-day accelerated partial breast irradiation using a MammoSite catheter (Benitez, et al. 2006; Berlin, Gjores, Ivarsson, Palmqvist, Thagg, & Thulesius, 1999; Borg et al., 2007; Dragun, Harper, Jenrette, Sinha, & Cole, 2007; Jeruss et al., 2006). Such novel radiotherapies targeting directly on the tumor site while avoiding scattering radiation to the axilla may have a role in reducing the risk of lymphedema in comparison to conventional radiotherapy. Research is needed to evaluate targeted radiotherapies in relation to lymphedema risk reduction. As a result, current surgical approaches for diagnosis of and treatment for breast cancer continue to make patients susceptible to the risk of lymphedema.

Besides unavoidable risk factors, such as breast surgery (mastectomy & lumpectomy), removal of lymph nodes (axillary lymph node dissection and sentinel lymph biopsy), presence of positive nodes, radiation and chemotherapy (Mak et al., 2008; Paskett et al., 2007), risk factors that can be managed or avoided are also identified, including obesity, weight gain after cancer treatment, minor upper extremity infections, injury or trauma to the affected side, overuse of the limb, and air travel (Johansson et al., 2002; Mak et al., 2008). Patient education is vital for implementing risk reduction behaviors targeting on such personal risk and triggering factors. In practice, many women treated for breast cancer have not received any information about lymphedema and risk reduction strategies (Fu et al., 2010; Ridner, 2006).

In a recent research on the effectiveness of lymphedema information provision among 136 breast cancer survivors (Fu et al., 2008; Fu et al., 2010), the researchers revealed that 43% percent of the participants reported that they did not receive any lymphedema information. Significantly fewer women who received lymphedema information reported swelling, heaviness, impaired shoulder mobility, seroma formation, and breast swelling. Regarding the most distressing symptom of arm swelling, 41% of patients who did not receive information reported arm swelling, comparing to 19% of those who received information. In terms of important cardinal symptoms of lymphedema, patients who did not receive information also reported significantly more symptoms of heaviness (27%), impaired shoulder mobility (32%), seroma formation (34%), breast swelling (32%), firmness/tightness (42%), numbness (39%), tenderness (54%), aching (36%), and stiffness (44%). In summary, patients who received lymphedema information reported significantly fewer symptoms than those who did not (t=3.03; p=0.00). With regard to risk reduction behaviors, patients who received information reported practicing significantly more risk reduction behaviors than those who did not (t=2.42, p=0.01). These behaviors included avoiding blood pressure, blood draws, and injections routinely done in the affected limb, wearing compression garments during air travel, treating minor injuries by washing and applying antibiotics, and most importantly, promoting lymph fluid drainage. In terms of cognitive outcome, patients who received information scored significantly higher in the knowledge test (t=0.49; p=0.00). The researchers developed a multiple regression model to assess the effects of provision of information on lymphedema related symptoms by taking into consideration of treatment-related risk factors. The results demonstrated that provision of information had significant reverse effect (**B**= -1.35; p<0.00) on lymphedema symptoms even taking into consideration of treatment-related risk factors. Together, provision of information and treatment-related risk factors account for 13% of variance (R^2= 0.13). After controlling for confounding factors, patient education remains an important predictor of lymphedema outcome.

Apparently, patient education is essential to promote risk reduction and early detection. In clinical practice, healthcare professionals could consider taking the initiative to provide adequate and accurate information and engage patients in supportive dialogues concerning lymphedema and risk reduction to improve patients' cognitive, behavior, and symptom outcomes. Healthcare professionals should equip themselves with lymphedema knowledge, including risk identification, early detection, and risk reduction strategies. Pretreatment education should focus on potential risk for lymphedema, brief review of the lymphatic system and pathophysiology of lymphedema, signs and symptoms of lymphedema, and risk reduction behaviors to reduce the risk from personal and triggering factors. Patients should be educated about the need to seek for professional help immediately if they begin to experience feelings of heaviness or tightness in at-risk limbs; or if they notice swelling in the affected area; or if the arm and/or at risk chest or truncal areas becomes hot or red. In the clinical settings, healthcare professionals could use the systematic assessment strategies to help patients to reduce the risk of lymphedema presented in Table 3.

5.2 Early detection

If undiagnosed or not treated effectively, lymphedema can progress into later stages of the condition resulting in a severe form of swelling known as elephantiasis (Figure 5). Early detection of lymphedema is believed to yield better patient outcomes to reduce the risk of the severe stage of lymphedema. To promote early detection, ongoing education should be conducted at each follow-up visit by reviewing the content of pretreatment education and encouraging the patient to report any signs and symptoms of lymphedema such as swelling, tightness, firmness, heaviness, aching, redness, rash, or increased temperature on the affected limb. As certain symptoms, such as tightness, and heaviness are associated with the onset of lymphedema (Armer et al., 2003; Cormier et al., 2009), it is important for healthcare providers to conduct a screening symptom assessment and refer breast cancer survivors with lymphedema to appropriate resources such as lymphedema therapy. (Table 3)

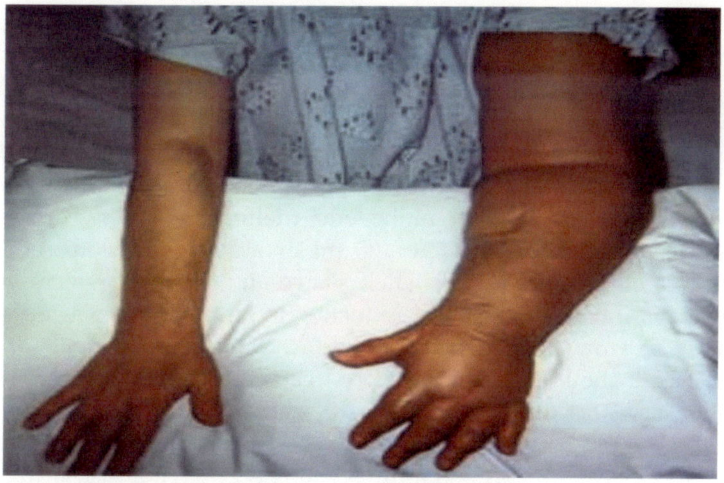

Fig. 6. Example of severe lymphedema known as elephantiasis

Risk Identification
- Ask the patient about history of cancer treatment
- Identify the affected or at-risk limb

Risk Reduction
- Recommend the patient use the *unaffected* side for blood pressure and blood work.
- If the patient had a bilateral mastectomy, suggest use the lower extremities for blood work and blood pressure.

Rationale: By using the unaffected side or lower extremities for blood draws and blood pressure, the patient will reduce the risk for infection, which lowers the risk of lymphedema.

Early Detection
- Use 3 questions to screen patients who might have developed lymphedema without awareness.

? Have you noticed any swelling in the affected hand, arm, breast, or trunk area?
? Have you experienced the feeling of heaviness, firmness, tightness in the affected side?
? Have you experienced any new discomfort in the affected side?

- Refer patient with early signs of symptoms to the certified lymphedema therapists.
- Assess the patients for signs and symptoms of infections (redness, tenderness, and pain). Administer antibiotics as needed.

Rationale:
- Early symptoms of lymphedema include slight swelling, heaviness, tightness, or firmness. It is important for nurses to assess these symptoms at each patient encounter, since early intervention can sometimes reverse lymphedema symptoms.
- It is important to assess signs and symptoms of infection (redness, tenderness, and pain). Infection, such as cellulitis, is the major predictor for lymphedema.

Table 3. Systematic Assessment Strategies for Lymphedema Risk Reduction

To promote early intervention, it is imperative to implement screening and measurement for early detection of breast cancer-related lymphedema. In a prospective observational study on 196 women with newly diagnosed breast cancer over a five year period (Stout et al., 2008), the women were measured using *infra-red Perometry* prior to their surgery and in three-month intervals following their surgery for up to one year. During that time, researchers were able to identify the development of subclinical lymphedema in 43 women (22%). The women with subclinical lymphedema (defined by the researchers as the limb volume change [LVC] of approximately 100 ml or a 3% LVC compared to the pre-op measure) were treated with an off-the- shelf sleeve and gauntlet, which was worn daily except during sleeping hours. Significant reduction in limb volume was observed that was similar to nearly the women's pre-surgical baseline value in all patients over an average period of 4.4 weeks. It should be noted that pre-treatment baseline measurement of limbs is essential, as this serves as the baseline data to which subsequent measurements can be compared. Healthcare professionals should use a cost-effective measuring method (such as circumferential arm measurement) and a time- and energy-saving measuring method (such as infra-red perometry) to monitor LVC in breast cancer survivors. Limb volume measurement should be conducted by the healthcare professionals who treat breast cancer and follow breast cancer survivors at each patient visit. In this way, patients with increased LV in the affected limb can be referred in a timely manner for further assessment and early intervention by specialists in lymphedema treatment.

6. Self-management for breast cancer-related lymphedema

Self-management for breast cancer-related lymphedema focuses on daily activities and strategies undertaken by breast cancer survivors to decrease the swelling, relieve symptoms, and prevent acute exacerbations and infections (Fu, 2005). As discussed previously, CDT requires patients to make a daily commitment by using external compression (sleeve, glove, wrap, bandage, or pump), performing remedial exercise, self-MLD and skin care (Davis, 1998; Rockson, et al. 1998). Self-management is essential for the success of the maintenance phase of the complete decongestive therapy (CDT) (Fu, 2010). Successful self-management of lymphedema also requires breast cancer survivors to initiate and maintain behaviors reduce triggering factors that can lead to severe lymphedema (Fu, 2005).

Limited research has been conducted on effective self-management of lymphedema. Very few exiting research are descriptive in nature yet the studies have delineated the difficulties and barriers that impede the effective self-management of lymphedema. A recent study revealed the major barriers to effective daily self-management include fatigue, lack of sufficient supporting system, insufficient financial resources, insufficient time, occupations involving manual laborious work, employers' misunderstanding, unsupportive working environment, fear of losing job (or stigma, embarrassment or discrimination), irregular working schedules, lack of clear or detailed instructions for self-care, lack of experience of organizing or following a schedule, and lack of experience of establishing or maintaining a routine (Fu, 2010). Currently, no research has been targeting on the identified barriers to promote self-management.

Breast cancer-related lymphedema is a chronic disease that, unlike other chronic illnesses such as arthritis or diabetes, receives little attention from healthcare professionals in clinical settings. To provide an emotional outlet for breast cancer survivors who may be concerned about developing lymphedema, healthcare professionals should consider asking the survivors if anyone has talked to them about lymphedema risk reduction practices, and if they are concerned about possibly developing lymphedema. For those with lymphedema, healthcare professionals may wish to ask about any problems they are having with swelling, skin integrity, or other problems or concerns they want to discuss related to their lymphedema. These activities, if done in any clinical setting, would begin to address the feelings of abandonment by healthcare professionals verbalized by many breast cancer survivors with lymphedema (Carter, 1997). Management of psychological distress and fatigue associated with lymphedema and self-management may require supportive services from healthcare professionals such as psychologists or conditioning experts (Fu, 2005; Ridner, 2005).

Similar to the self-management for other chronic illnesses, healthcare professionals have a significant role in ensuring effective self-management of lymphedema by motivating breast cancer survivors. Some cognitive, psychological, and social strategies can help breast cancer survivors to promote and maintain self-management behaviors (Fu, 2004). Cognitive strategies refer to breast cancer survivors' ability to understand the need for change of behaviors to implement daily self-management activities and ability to identify and overcome barriers in carrying out such activities. Patient education is the optimal way to enhance breast cancer survivors' knowledge and provide relevant resources.

Psychological strategies include those that help breast cancer survivors set goals for their lymphedema management and motivate them to continue their daily management activities. Fu (2005) identifies four major intentions undertaken by breast cancer survivors to promote effective daily lymphedema management: keeping in mind the consequences, preventing lymphedema from getting worse, getting ready to live with lymphedema, and integrating the care of lymphedema into daily life. The four intentions reveal in detail the way in which breast cancer survivors structure their lives to manage lymphedema daily. Healthcare professionals are in the best position to identify breast cancer survivors' individual needs by assessing the presence or absence of the intentions. In another recent study (Fu, 2010), the researcher described how breast cancer survivors actively and creatively structured their lives to make lymphedema self-management feasible by making conscious decisions about new-fangled limitations, making daily care feasible, and incorporating lymphedema care into daily routine. The study also identified effective and ineffective strategies and barriers to fulfill the intentions of self management (Table 4). Research is needed to develop interventions to test the identified effective strategies for self-management of lymphedema.

Social strategies focus on providing resources or support groups to externally enhance breast cancer survivors' motivation to continue self-management to maintain LV and deal with physical symptoms as well as psychological distress and social anxiety. Internal and external resources, such as programs about lymphedema treatment and reliable internet websites, should be given to breast cancer survivors. Providing social support helps mitigate breast cancer survivors' sense of being singled-out, a perspective that was vividly described by a breast cancer survivors with five years of lymphedema, "You feel that you are on this little island by yourself and just struggling because there is no one else around who knows what lymphedema is" (Fu, 2003, p. 188). Support group in which women can feel free to share their success stories about lymphedema management and the ways of overcoming

Making Self Management Feasible			
Intentions	**Effective Strategies**	**Barriers to the strategy**	**Ineffective Strategies**
Making Conscious Decisions about New-fangled Limitations	• Giving up • Letting go • Asking for help • Paying for help • Using the unaffected limb	• Lack of sufficient supporting system of family, friends, and coworkers • Unsupportive working environment • Employers' misunderstanding • Insufficient financial resources • Occupations involving manual laborious work • Impatience	• Ignoring • Forgetting • Neglecting
Making daily Care Feasible	• Wearing daytime compressive garments as much as possible • Using *Easy Slide* or other device to help putting on the compression sleeve • Wrapping the affected arm during nighttime • Using rubber gloves to protect the compression gloves from getting dirty • Performing exercise and massage if time and physical stamina allow • Getting an easy access to the things needed for lymphedema care • Spacing out the household chores • Having someone help • Wearing protective gloves for dish washing, cleaning, and gardening • Using food processor to cut food	• Lack of clear or detailed instructions • Insufficient time • Insufficient financial resources • Insufficient qualified therapists • Fatigue • Fear of losing job, stigma, embarrassment or discrimination • Occupations involving manual laborious work • Employers' misunderstanding • Unsupportive working environment • Lack of sufficient supporting system	• Trying to do all that you were told
Incorporating Lymphedema Care into Daily Routine	• Establishing and sustaining a daily routine • Foreseeing the changes in life • Readjusting to the established routine	• Lack of experience of organizing or following a schedule • Lack of experience of establishing or maintaining a routine • Insufficient time • Irregular working schedules • Fatigue • Being a good wife and loving mother	• Following an irregular schedule

Table 4. Intentions, Effective strategies, Barriers and Ineffective Strategies (Adapted from: Fu, M.R. (2010). Cancer Survivors' views of lymphoedema management. *Journal of Lymphoedema, 5*(2), 39-48.)

barriers is an effective way to provide social support (Fu, 2005). Well-designed support groups can also enhance skills for effective lymphedema management through group practice of certain skills such as easier ways of putting on a compression garment, applying bandage or wraps, and performing self-MLD. Group practice allows the opportunity not only for building a community to further promote breast cancer survivors' sense of belongingness, but also for transforming routine lymphedema management activities into fun activities that may elicit interest and enjoyment to sustain the women's motivation. The lifetime commitment to manage lymphedema requires time and effort by both breast cancer survivors and healthcare professionals to insure that quality life is not profoundly impacted.

7. Strategies for personal and family-level care

7.1 Individual-level psychosocial impacts

It has been well documented that psychological health can be impacted by changes in physical appearance and limitations created by lymphedema (e.g., Petrek et al., 2001; Radina & Armer, 2001, 2004; Thomas-MacLean et al., 2005). This includes both mental health concerns and the ways in which patients cope with the physical limitations brought on my breast cancer-related lymphedema in their daily lives.

7.1.1 Mental health concerns

In addition to the physical limitations of breast cancer-related lymphedema, patients are also subject to potential psychosocial problems including depression, anxiety, poor adjustment to illness, and low self esteem (Maunsell, Brisson, & Deschenes, 1993; Thomas-MacLean et al., 2005). Chachaj and collegues (2010) found that there were several factors that contributed to patients' experiences of negative psychosocial outcomes. These included "pain in the upper limb (mainly shoulder and arm), pain in operated breast, difficulties with arm movement, localization of lymphedema within the hand or in operated breast, a history of dermatolymphangitis and of receiving chemotherapy"(p. Vassard and colleagues (2010) explored the psychosocial outcomes of patients engaged in post-breast cancer surgery rehabilitation. They found that compared with patients who did not develop lymphedema, those with lymphedema reported a greater impact on their psychological well-being. Specifically, patients with breast cancer-related lymphedema were more likely to report lower overall quality of life and perceiving themselves to be in poorer health. These findings are similar to those reported by Heiney and colleagues (2007) who found that both physical and social aspects of quality of life were impacted by breast cancer-related lymphedema. Researchers have also found that the degree to which patients experience negative impacts on their mental health and quality of life is correlated with the severity of the lymphedema symptoms and the degree to which these symptoms are viewed as distressful (Erickson et al., 2001; Kornblith, Herndon, Weiss, Zhang, Zuckerman, Rosenberg et al., 2003). Similarly, Ridner (2005) found that patients with breast cancer-related lymphedema reported higher levels of emotional distress and reduced body confidence then those without lymphedema. Certainly this finding of reduced body confidence has implications for patients' self-esteem as well as sexual intimacy. With regard to addressing psychosocial problems in this population, Hamilton, Miedema, MacIntyre, & Easley, 2011) investigated the use of a positive self-talk intervention. Their findings suggest that such interventions may have a positive impact on patients' coping skills. They argue that further investigations are needed to determine appropriate psychological interventions that positively impact such mental health concerns as anxiety and depression among patients with breast cancer-related lymphedema.

7.1.2 Coping with physical limitations in daily life

Lymphedema can impose limitations on women's lives in terms of their ability to participate in normal, daily activities (Radina & Armer, 2001; Ridner, 2002). Radina (2009) found that women with breast cancer-related lymphedema experienced a heightened sense of awareness and caution concerning their physical activities, as well as a sense of frustration with the limitations they faced as a result of breast cancer-related lymphedema. At the same time, these women also must engage in time consuming self-care, as described above, in order to reduce and control the swelling associated with lymphedema (e.g., manual lymph draining, CDT). Not only are some of these treatments restricting in terms of range of motion, but they also require the patient to set aside time during the day to perform them and to potentially ask others (i.e., family members) for help. The patient must also avoid getting any wrappings wet and therefore must remove the wrapping and rewrap the arm for bathing or other water activities (e.g., swimming, washing dishes). Lastly, because the compression sleeve is so expensive and must be washed by hand everyday, the patient must be careful not to stain or otherwise damage the sleeve (Casley-Smith, 1992).

7.2 Family/interpersonal relationship-level psychosocial impacts

Given the increasing large population of women living as breast cancer survivors and the understanding that breast cancer impacts the entire family, not just the patient/survivor (Baider, Cooper, & Kaplan De-Nour, 2000; Veach, Nicholas, & Barton, 2002), a growing number of families may be facing the need to navigate survivorship as well. At the same time, given that as many as 40% of women who have gone through breast cancer treatment may develop breast-cancer related lymphedema, there is also a growing number of families who are not only needing to cope with cancer survivorship in general but also coping daily with the chronic condition of lymphedema.

The study of breast cancer survivorship in general has largely centered on the experiences of breast cancer patients and has failed to sufficiently consider the impact that breast cancer diagnosis and treatment can have on family members and family life. The majority of work that considers family members is focused on breast cancer patients' relationships with husbands and young children (e.g., Northouse, Laten, & Reddy, 1995; Radina, 2009; Radina & Armer, 2001; 2004, Radina, Watson, & Faubert, 2009; Rees & Bath, 2000) and the individual quality of life of patients and their family members in the context of breast cancer (e.g., Kim & Given, 2008; Northouse et al., 2002). Only recently have researchers focused attention on how family functioning and adaptation can influence the lives of breast cancer patients and survivors (e.g., Mallinger, Griggs, & Shields, 2006; Radina, 2009; Radina & Armer, 2001; 2004; Radina et al., 2009). The evolution of empirically based understanding of how cancer in general impacts the family continues to evolve. The limited research that explores family dynamics in the context of breast cancer focuses on issues such as participation in treatment decision making (Lacey, 2002; Raveis & Pretter, 2004), family communication patterns both prior to and after the breast cancer diagnosis (Forest, Plumb,

Ziebland, & Stein, 2009; Mallinger et al., 2006), and the family's role as either a supportive or distressing unit (Alfano & Roland, 2006; Spencer et al., 1999). Here we review the research that has been conducted that investigates the specific ways in which breast cancer patients with lymphedema experience their family and interpersonal lives with regard to family work, family play, and sexual intimacy with significant romantic others. We conclude by exploring a theory of health-related family quality of life and how it might be applied to families coping with breast cancer-related lymphedema.

7.2.1 Family work and family play

The daily lives and rhythms of families include both getting the work of the family completed (i.e., housework) and the maintenance of family relationships (i.e., spending quality time together). Researchers have shown that both aspects of family functioning can be impacted by the onset and continued care required of breast cancer-related lymphedema (Radina, 2009; Radina & Armer 2001; 2004). That is, the physical limitations and psychosocial difficulties experienced by women with lymphedema frequently require the individual and her family members to renegotiate family roles and modify how they function as a unit (Radina & Armer, 2001; 2004). With regard to family work, this may include a redistribution of household responsibilities (i.e., asking an adult son to run the vacuum or employing a maid service to do the heavy cleaning) or the modification of how and if such responsibilities are undertaken (i.e., lowering standards of household cleanliness, learning to use the other arm to sweep the kitchen floor) (Radina & Armer, 2001). Women at-risk for developing breast cancer-related lymphedema have been shown to struggle with balancing the needs of others (e.g., family members) with their own needs for self-care that are aimed at reducing their risk of developing or exacerbating breast cancer-related lymphedema (Radina, Armer, & Stewart, under review). Gilligan and others (e.g., Jack, 1991; Ruddick, 1989) have argued that women are socialized within family and community life to embrace this concept of self-sacrifice in the service of others. Caring for others, and doing so in an unselfish way or at the expense of one's own needs, is the currency that women are socialized to deal with in order to create and maintain relationships with others (Jack, 1991). The role women often assume in family life requires some degree of self-sacrifice in order to manage the household and take care of family members (Mederer, 1993), including paid work outside the home. In this sense, what gets put on hold are activities like personal care, medication, exercise, or other activities that are largely for the benefit of the woman alone and not explicitly benefiting the family as a whole or individual family members. Radina and colleagues (under review) found that women at-risk for developing breast cancer-related lymphedema struggled with making their self-care a priority despite being enrolled in an intervention study aimed at teaching them techniques for self-care to reduce their risk of developing breast cancer-related lymphedema. Often the major barrier to self-care was the pull they felt to put others' needs first. Consistent with Ridner, Dietrich, and Kidd (2011) of women diagnosed with lymphedema, Radina et al. (under review) found that these women at-risk for developing lymphedema struggled with finding the time in their daily lives to engage in self-care. Radina and colleagues' findings highlight the important role that social contexts (e.g., family life, gendered expectations) can play as a factor in personal care for breast cancer survivors.

Radina (2009) found that for some women with breast cancer-related lymphedema, lifestyle modifications extend beyond daily activities such as dressing, bathing, cooking, and housekeeping into the realm of leisure. When it comes to leisure activities, wives and mothers who are often responsible for family management, are likely to be the ones creating time and space for other family members' independent leisure activities (e.g., backing cupcakes for her son's football team party, driving children to music lessons). Because of these other responsibilities, women's independent leisure is often sacrificed so that they can accomplish these other tasks for their families (Henderson, Bialeschki, Shaw, & Freysinger, 1999).

For women, their own participation in leisure activities in general, whether engaged in individually or with their families, may act as a buffer against stressful life events such as breast cancer and breast cancer-related lymphedema (Pondé & Santana, 2000). Thus, the continued participation of women with lymphedema in leisure activities appears valuable for sustaining their quality of life after breast cancer treatment. At the same time, family leisure is important for understanding family functioning (Zabriski & McCormick, 2001), particularly in the context of chronic health conditions and health-related disabilities (Jo, Kosciulek, Huh, & Holecek, 2004). Radina (2009) found that breast cancer-related lymphedema can create serious limitations that can impact both family functioning and participation in leisure.

Family interaction in the context of leisure enhances the family's ability to remain stable (Orthner & Mancini, 1990). In fact, researchers have demonstrated that there is a positive relationship between family leisure engagement, family satisfaction, and family quality of life (Zabriskie & McCormick, 2003). The Core and Balance Model of Family Leisure Functioning (Zabriskie, 2000; Zabriskie & McCormick, 2001) suggests that family adaptability (i.e., the family's ability to be flexible and change), cohesion (i.e., closeness, emotional bonding), and communication are facilitated through family members' joint engagement in family-based leisure activities (Zabriskie & McCormick, 2001). These can include both core and balance leisure activities. Core leisure activities are "common everyday, low-cost, relatively accessible, and often home-based activities that families do frequently" (Zabriskie & McCormick, 2003, p. 168) including such activities as playing a game, e-mailing or instant messaging with family members, and making/eating dinner together (Zabriskie & McCormick, 2001). Core leisure activities tend to be associated with the maintenance of family cohesion and thus families who perceived themselves as having high levels of emotional closeness report engaging in more core leisure activities (Zabriskie, McCormick, & Austin, 2001). Balance leisure activities are "less common, less frequent, more out of the ordinary, and usually not home based thus providing novel experiences" (Zabriskie & McCormick, 2003, p. 168) including such activities as family travel, family reunions, and special family events (Zabriskie & McCormick, 2001). Balance activities tend to be associated with maintaining family adaptability (Zabriskie et al., 2001). According to the Core and Balance Model, in order to have healthier family functioning that results from increased levels of family communication, families should participate in both core and balance activities that enhance both family cohesion and adaptability (Zabriskie & McCormick, 2003).

The role that family leisure plays generally also applies to families in which there is a chronically ill or disabled member (i.e., lymphedema). For such families participating in shared leisure time is associated with enhanced family communication and stability (Guerin & Dattilo, 2001). For individuals with disabilities, the benefits of leisure activities (e.g., increases in self-confidence, social networks, and one's sense of accomplishment and satisfaction) have been well-established (Jo et al., 2004; Lloyd, King, Lampe, & McDougall, 2001). Despite this relationship, families with a disabled member are less likely to participate in balance leisure activities (38%) compared to families without a member with a disability (52%; Jo et al., 2004).

Radina (2009) found that women with breast cancer-related lymphedema approached their participation in family leisure activities in two ways. The first involved continued participation in family leisure activities but with extra care (e.g., purchasing light weight hiking equipment) or being creative about how they participated (e.g., becoming the scout troop treasurer rather than accompanying children on back packing trips). The second strategy involved withdrawing from family activities that according to the Core and Balance Model (Zabriskie et al., 2001) could jeopardize overall levels of family functioning by eliminating opportunities for building or improving family adaptability, cohesion, or communication.

7.2.2 Sexuality and intimacy

Sexuality can be examined as an interaction of biological, psychological, and social domains of life (Lindau, Laumann, Levinson, & Waite, 2003; National Institute on Aging, 2005). How individuals feel about themselves as sexual beings is impacted by a combination of all three of these areas. As women with breast cancer-related lymphedema have already faced breast cancer, their feelings about sexuality and intimacy are intertwined with their breast cancer and lymphedema experiences. Thus, it may not be possible to completely distinguish between body image issues, feelings of sexuality, and the impact on sexual relationships brought about by breast cancer and those resulting from lymphedema.

Researchers have explored the impact of breast cancer on sexuality and sexual relationships (e.g., Henson, 2002). This work has included investigations into the impact of breast cancer and its treatment on hormones and sexual functioning, attitudes of a romantic partner, the impact of fatigue brought about by treatment on sexual relationships, and how an altered body image resulting from (breast) cancer can impact one's sexuality and sexual relationships (Gould, Grassau, Manthorne, Gray, & Fitch, 2006). Research also have focused on how there tends to be a lack of information on how breast cancer and its treatment can impact sexuality that is provided to breast cancer patient and their partners (Gould et al., 2006; Henson, 2002).

With breast cancer-related lymphedema, women may experience changes in their appearance as well as pain and physical limitations due to swelling (Passik & McDonald, 1998). As sexuality is connected to a woman's feelings about herself and her body, not only the experience of breast cancer, but also the development of lymphedema can have a serious impact on her views of herself as sexual and her willingness to be physical with a partner. Having survived breast cancer to now have to contend with breast cancer-related lymphedema can be seen "as a secondary blow to their physical and emotional well-being," which includes their intimate relationships with others (Passik and McDonald, 1998, p. 2818). Research (e.g., Koch et al., 2005; Radina, Watson, & Faubert, 2009; Wiederman &

Hurst, 1997) has highlighted the negative ways in which women with breast-cancer related lymphedema feel about their bodies and how these feeling can take away from their desire to engage in sexual activity with a partner. Radina et al (2009) and Gould et al. (2006) found that the disfiguring aspects of breast cancer as well as breast cancer-related lymphedema made women feel unattractive and self-conscious about their bodies. Radina et al (2009) also found that women with breast-cancer related lymphedema expressed feeling that current or future sexual partners might not find them sexy because of the lymphedema and/or the compression garments that they need to be wear to treat their conditions.

There are numerous studies that explore the connection of sexual satisfaction, self or body image, and physical disability (e.g., Kedde & van Berlo, 2006; Taleporos, Dip, & McCabe, 2002; Galvin, 2005). Lymphedema can be not only be a condition with disfiguring effects but also debilitating ones. Galvin (2005) studied narratives of disabled people with a diverse range of disability and impairment. Based on this research, the term "disabled identity" emerged to reflect a self-perception that is affected by appearance, sexuality, and the negative attitudes of others. Shame and fear of rejection were related to reactions from others for those whose impairment was evident or visible. Feelings of loss of attractiveness, negative reactions of others, and internalized societal messages about the asexuality of disabled people contributed to feelings of loss of sexuality in many of the narratives (Galvin, 2005). Although not a "disability," because of the disfiguring and disabling aspects of the condition of lymphedema, the "disabled identity," which is impacted by an internalization of how others view this condition, can negatively impact sexuality and one's desire to be sexual with others.

7.2.3 Family quality of life

Radina and Armer (2004) explored outcomes for women with breast cancer-related lymphedema within the context of their families using the Resiliency Model of Family Stress, Adjustment, and Adaptation (M. A. McCubbin & H. I. McCubbin, 1996). They found instances where participants described themselves and their families as either adjusting (i.e., making small changes in family patterns of functioning in order to cope with lymphedema), adapting (i.e., making major changes in family patterns of functioning in order to cope with lymphedema), or living in crisis. Specifically, those families who were resilient had shared perception of the limitations brought on by lymphedema as being manageable and something that could be incorporated into patterns of daily living. At the same time, the more resilient families pulled together as a family to make necessary changes (e.g., the entire family focusing on the lymphedema and supporting the patient, the patient or her spouse changing jobs, using humor and inside jokes). The ingenuity and perseverance demonstrated by resilient families suggest that the families of women with breast cancer-related lymphedema can be resilient in coping with lymphedema.

One way to think about family life in the context of breast cancer-related lymphedema is to consider the concept of health-related family quality of life. Health-related family quality of life refers to a state of being for families in the context of one or more family members' illnesses as well as the processes that families use to cope. Below I provide an overview of a theory of Health-Related Family Quality of Life whose purpose is to provide a model of understanding what family quality of life is within the specific context of breast cancer and, by extension, breast cancer-related lymphedema. Below the assumptions, concepts, and propositions of this theory of Health-Related Family Quality of Life are presented.

The first assumption is that families are made up of multiple actors who interact based on established patterns of functioning that are governed by rules that can be both explicit and implicit (Bigner, 1998). Second, new or revised patterns of functioning can result when a stressor (e.g., breast cancer) is encountered by the family (M. A. McCubbin & H. I., McCubbin, 1991; 1996; Olson, Lavee, & McCubbin, 1988). Third, the introduction of that stressor to the family allows for established patterns of functioning to become apparent when they otherwise might not be (Ingoldsby, Smith, & Miller, 2004; Molassiotis, 1997). Fourth, quality of family life is subjective and situation-dependent (McCabe et al., 2008).

As is detailed in Figure 5, the theory of Health-Related Family Quality of Life is made up of three overarching concepts: emotional closeness, family self-efficacy, and family functioning. *Emotional closeness* includes feelings of psychological or affectional closeness toward and/or between family members as well as such feelings toward the family as a unit (Bengtson, 1991; Poston et al., 2003). At the same time, the concept of emotional closeness also includes family communication as a way of facilitating and demonstrating closeness (Bigner, 1998; M. A. McCubbin & H. I., McCubbin, 1991; 1996; Poston et al., 2003). Family communication is made up of family members' feelings regarding the quality, quantity, frequency, and content of this communication (Bengston, 1991). Lastly, the concept of emotional closeness also includes social support-both among family members and for the family as a unit from those outside the family. Social support can also be considered a resource that the family uses in managing the quality of their family life (Hill, 1949; Patterson, 2002; Poston et al., 2003). *Family Self-Efficacy* refers to the families meaning-making about themselves as a unit and the illness (i.e., sense of coherence), in this case breast cancer. Hill (1949) and others (e.g., Anderson, 1993; Caplan, 1987; McCabe et al., 2008) point to the importance of appraisal of stressors as essential to understanding how the stressor will be handled. That is, if a family considers the stressor to be catastrophic, this may have a negative influence on family quality of life in that it may be seen as irrevocable damaged. As part of this meaning-making, family self-efficacy includes family members' sense of both family strengths (Smith-Bird & Turnbull, 2005) and their ability to cope with challenges (i.e., possibly based on the family's history of how they face challenges and their success with overcoming them; Hill, 1949; M. A. McCubbin & H. I., McCubbin, 1991; 1996; Mellon & Northouse, 2001; Patterson, 2002). Lastly, *Family Functioning* consists of family members' roles and responsibilities (e.g., family care, daily activities, getting help) as well as their satisfaction with how well the family meets individual and family unit needs (Bigner, 1998; Ingoldsby et al., 2004; Park et al., 2003; Rettig & Leichtentritt, 1999).

The theory of Health-Related Family Quality of Life offers three propositions about how health-related family quality of life functions. First, the theory of Health-Related Family Quality of Life is based on family members' perceptions of emotional closeness, family efficacy, and satisfaction with needs being met. Second, changes in family quality of life are based on perceptions of changes in emotional closeness, family self-efficacy, and patterns of functioning. Third, emotional closeness and family self-efficacy are considered resources that families utilize when faced with a stressor.

The application of the theory of Health-Related Family Quality of Life sheds light on the varying factors that can contribute to how a family reacts to and copes with breast cancer-related lymphedema. For some families these factors may already be working well meaning that they will be predisposed to maintain a positive health-related quality of life in the context of breast cancer-related lymphedema. Others, however, may need coaching from trained professionals in order to enhance or improve their health-related quality of life. The professionals need not be family counselors, family life educators, or social works alone. Others, including health care professionals, should be aware of the impact breast cancer-related lymphedema can have on family quality of life so that they may also help both patients and their family members thrive.

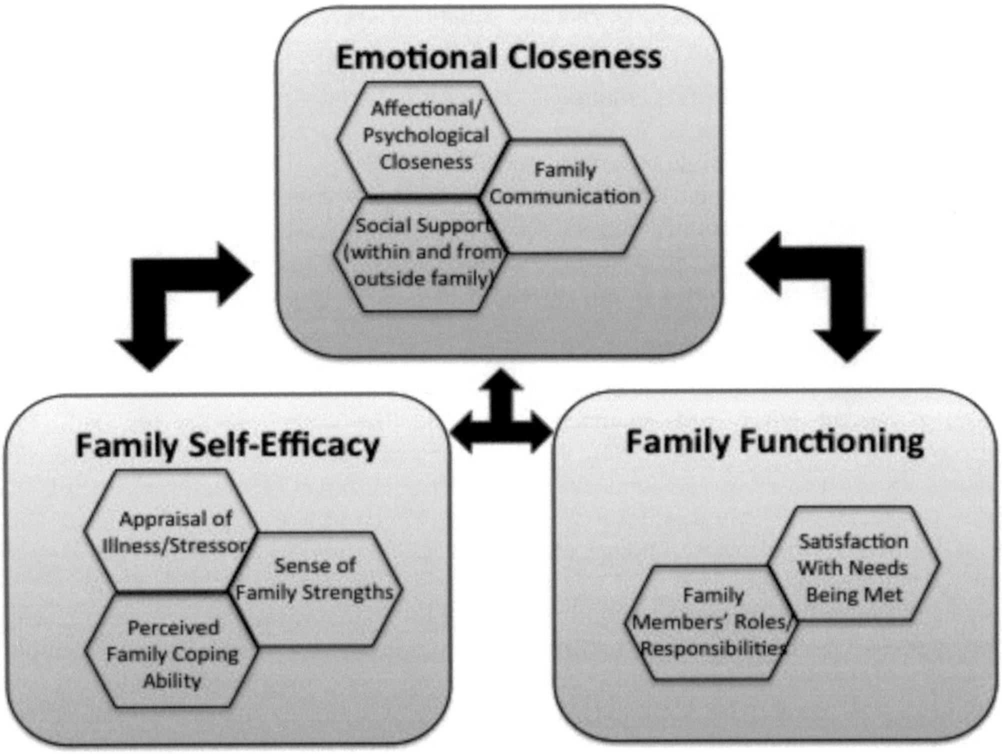

Fig. 7. Theory of Health-Related Family Quality of Life

8. Conclusion

Up to 40% of breast cancer patients are likely to develop breast cancer-related lymphedema. Thus, patients and their family members must learned to not only prepare for but cope with this often disabling chronic condition. Thus, the focus of this chapter was on patient (and family member/caregiver) education regarding strategies for early detection, risk reduction, and management/self-care and the individual and family level psychosocial impacts of coping with breast cancer-related lymphedema. The topics covered in this chapter were chosen with the intention of informing readers (e.g., physicians, nursing, social workers, family therapists, family life educators, and others who work with patients and their families) about the needs of patients and their family members and provide strategies to meet the needs of patients and families. In this way, wide ranging support for patients and their family members would be encouraged and implemented throughout the trajectory of patient care.

9. References

Ahmed, R. L., Thomas, W., Yee, D., & Schmitz, K. H. (2006). Randomized controlled trial of weight training and lymphedema in breast cancer survivors. *Journal of Clinical Oncoogy,* 24(18):2765-2772.

Alfano, C.M., & Roland, J.H. (2006). Recovery issues in cancer survivorship: A new challenge for supportive care. *Cancer Journal, 12*(5), 432-43

American Cancer Society. (2010). *Cancer facts & figures 2010.* Atlanta, GA: American Cancer Society. Retrieved on-line July 26, 2010: http://www.cancer.org/acs/groups/content/@nho/documents/document/acspc-024113.pdf

American Cancer Society. (2007). *Global Cancer Facts & Figures.* Atlanta, GA: Author.

Anderson, K.E.H. (1993). The relative contribution to illness stress and family system variables to family quality of life during early chronic illness. *Dissertation Abstracts International, 54*(06), 2991.

Armer, J., Fu, M.R., Wainstock, J.M., Zagar, E., & Jacobs, L.K. (2004). Lymphedema following breast cancer treatment, including sentinel lymph node biopsy. *Lymphology, 37,* 73-91.

Armer, J. M., Radina, M. E., Porock, D., & Culbertson, S. D. (2003). Predicting breast cancer-related lymphedema using self- reported symptoms. *Nursing Research, 52*(6), 370-379.

Armer, J.M., & Stewart, B.R. (2005). A comparison of four diagnostic criteria for lymphedema in a post-breast cancer population. *Lymphatic Research & Biology, 3*(4), 208-217.

Armer, J. M., Stewart, B. R., & Shook, R. P. (2009). 30-month post-breast cancer treatment lymphoedema. *Journal of Lymphoedema, 4*(1), 14-18.

Armer, J. M., & Whitman, M. (2002). The problem of lymphedema following breast cancer treatment: Prevalence, symptoms, & self-management. *Lymphology, 35 (suppl),* 153-159.

Badger, C., Preston, N., Seers, K., Mortimer, P. (2004). Benzo-pyrones for reducing and controlling lymphoedema of the limbs. *Cochrane Database System Review, (2)*:CD003140.

Beaulac, S. M., McNair, L. A., Scott, T. E., LaMorte, W. W., & Kavanah, M. T. (2002). Lymphedema and quality of life in survivors of early-stage breast cancer. *Archives of Surgery, 137,* 1253-1257.

Bengston, V.L., & Roberts, R.E.L. (1991). Intergenerational solidarity in families: An example of formal theory construction. *Journal of Marriage and the Family, 53,* 856-870.

Benitez, P.R., Streeter, O., Vicini, F., Mehta, V., Quiet, C., Kuske, R., et al. (2006). Preliminary results and evaluation of MammoSite balloon brachytherapy for partial breast irradiation for pure ductal carcinoma in situ: a phase II clinical study. *American Journal of Surgery, 192*(4), 427-33.

Berlin, E., Gjores, J. E., Ivarsson, C., Palmqvist, I., Thagg, G., & Thulesius, O. (1999). Postmastectomy lymphedema:

Treatment and a five-year follow-up study. *International Angiology: A Journal of the International Union of Angiology, 18*(4), 294-298.

Bigner, J.J. (1998). *Parent-child relations: An introduction to parenting*. Upper Saddle River, NJ: Merrill.

Boneti, C., Korourian, S., Bland, K., Cox, K., Adkins, L.L., Henry-Tillman, R.S., Klimberg, V.S. (2008). Axillary reverse mapping: mapping and preserving arm lymphatics may be important in preventing lymphedema during sentinel lymph node biopsy. *Journal of the American College of Surgeons, 206*(5), 1038-42.

Borg, M., Yeoh, E., Bochner, M., Butters, J., van Doorn, T., Farshid, G., et al. (2007). Feasibility study on the MammoSite in early-stage breast cancer: initial experience. *Australasian Radiology, 51*(1), 53-61.

Boris, M., Weidorf, S., & Lasinski, B. (1997). Persistence of lymphedema reduction after noninvasive complex lymphedema therapy. *Oncology, 11*(1), 99-114.

Brennan, M.J., & Miller, L.T. (1998). Overview of treatment options and review of the current role and use of compression garments, intermittent pumps, and exercise in the management of lymphedema. *Cancer, 83*(12 Suppl American), 2821-2827.

Bruns, F., Micke, O., Bremer, M. (2003). Current status of selenium and other treatments for secondary lymphedema. *Journal of Support Oncology, 1*(2):121-130.

Callaway, C.W., Chumlea,W.C., Bouchard, C., Himes, J.H., Lohman, T.G., Martin, A.D., et al. (1988). Circumferences. In T.G Lohman, A.F. Roche, & R. Martorell (Eds.), *Anthropometric standardization reference manual,* (pp. 39-51). Champaign, IL: Human Kinetics Books.

Cambria, R.A., Gloviczki, P., Naessens, J.M., Wahner, H.W. (1993). Noninvasive evaluation of the lymphatic system with lymphoscintigraphy: a prospective, semiquantitative analysis in 386 extremities. *Journal of Vasular Surgery, 18*(5):773-782.

Campisi C, Boccardo F, Zilli A, et al. Long-term results after lymphatic-venous anastomoses for the treatment of obstructive lymphedema. Microsurgery. 2001;21:135–9.

Caplan, K.C. (1987). Definitions and dimensions of quality of life. In N. K. Aaronson & J. Beckmann (Eds.), *The quality of life of cancer patients*, (p. 1-9). New York, NY: Raven.

Casley-Smith, J. R. (1992). Modern treatment of lymphoedema. *Modern Medicine of Australia, 35*(5), 70-83.

Chachaj, A., Małyszczak, K., Pyszel, K., Lukas, J., Tarkowski, R., Pudełko, M., Andrzejak, R., & Szuba, A. (2010). Physical and psychological impairments of women with upper limb lymphedema following breast cancer treatment. *Psycho- oncology, 19*(3), 299-305.

Cormier, J.N., Rourke, L., Crosby, M., Chang, D., Armer, J. (2011). The Surgical Treatment of Lymphedema: A Systematic Review of the Contemporary Literature (2004-2010). Annals of Surgical Oncology, DOI 10.1245/s10434-011-2017-4

Cormier, J.N., Xing, Y., Zaniletti, I., Askew, R.L., Stewart, B.R., Armer, J.M. (2009). Minimal limb volume change has a significant impact on breast cancer survivors. *Lymphology, 42*, 161-175.

Cornish, B.H., Chapman, M., Hirst, C., Mirolo, B., Bunce, I.H., Ward, L.C., et al. (2001). Early diagnosis of lymphedema using multiple frequency bioimpedance. *Lymphology, 34*(1), 2-11.

Coster, S., Poole, K., & Fallowfield, L. J. (2001). The validation of a quality of life scale to assess the impact of arm morbidity in breast cancer patients post-operatively. *Breast Cancer Research and Treatment, 68*(3), 273-282.

Davis S. (1998). Lymphedema following breast cancer treatment. *Radiologic Technology, 70*(1), 42-56.

Disa, J. J., & Petrek, J. (2001). Rehabilitation after treatment for cancer of the breast. In V. T. DeVita, Jr., S. Hellman & S. A. Rosenberg (Eds.), *CANCER Principles and Practice of Oncology* (6th edition ed., pp. 1717-1726). Philadelphia: Lippincott, Williams & Wilkins.

Dragun, A.E., Harper, J.L., Jenrette, J.M., Sinha, D., & Cole, D.J. (2007). Predictors of cosmetic outcome following MammoSite breast brachytherapy: A single-institution experience of 100 patients with two years of follow-up. *International Journal of Radiation Oncology, Biology, Physics, 68*(2), 354-358.

Enderling, H., Anderson, A.R., Chaplain, M.A., Munro, A.J., & Vaidya, J.S. (2006). Mathematical modeling of radiotherapy: Strategies for early breast cancer. *Journal of Theoretical Biology, 241,* 158-171.

Erickson, V.S., Pearson, M.L., Ganz, P.A., Adams, J., Kahn, K.L. (2001). Arm edema in breast cancer patients. *Journal of National Cancer Institute*, 93(2):96-111.

Ferlay, J., Bray, F., Pisani, P., & Parkin, D. M. (2004). *GLOBOCAN 2002: Cancer Incidence, Mortality and Prevalence Worldwide*. Lyon, France: IARCPress.

Foeldi, M. Foeldi, E, Clodius, L., & Neu, H. (2003). Complications of lymphedema. In M. Foeldi, E. Foeldi, & S. Kubik (Eds). *Textbook of lymphology for physicians and lymphedema* therapists (pp. 267-275). Munchen: Urban & Fischer Verlag: Elsevier GmbH. English text revised by Biotext LLC, San Francisco, CA.

Forest, G., Plumb, C., Ziebland, S., & Stein, A. (2009). Breast cancer in young families: A qualitative interview study of fathers and their role and communication with their children following the diagnosis of maternal breast cancer. *Psycho-oncology, 18*(1), 96-103.

Fu, M.R. & Rosedale, M. (2009). Breast Cancer Survivors' Experience of Lymphedema Related Symptoms. *Journal of Pain and Symptom Management, 38*(6), 849-59. PMID: 19819668. NIHMS[142640]

Fu, M.R. (2003). *Managing lymphedema in breast cancer survivors*. Doctoral Dissertation, Research, University of Missouri- Columbia.

Fu, M.R. (2004). Post-breast cancer lymphedema and management. *Recent Advances: Research Updates, 5*(1), 125-138.

Fu, M.R. (2005). Breast cancer survivors' intentions of managing lymphedema. *Cancer Nursing, 28*(6), 446-457.

Fu, M.R., Axelrod, D. & Haber, J. (2008). Breast Cancer-Related Lymphedema: Information, Symptoms, and Risk Reduction Behaviors. *Journal of Nursing Scholarship, 40*(4), 341-348.

Fu, M.R., Chen, C., Haber, J., Guth, A. & Axelrod, D. (2010). The Effect of Providing Information about Lymphedema on the Cognitive and Symptom Outcomes of Breast Cancer Survivors. *Annals of Surgical Oncology, 17*(7),1847-53. Epub 2010 Feb 6.PMID: 20140528. DOI 10.1245/s10434-010-0941-3

Fu, M.R. (2010). Cancer Survivors' views of lymphoedema management. *Journal of Lymphoedema, 5*(2), 39-48.

Galvin, R. D. (2005). Researching the disabled identity: Contextualising the identity transformations which accompany the onset of impairment. *Sociology of Health & Illness, 27,* 393-413.

Geller, B. M., Vacek, P. M., O'Brien, P., & Secker-Walker, R. H. (2003). Factors associated with arm swelling after breast cancer surgery. *Journal of Women's Health, 12*(9), 921-930.

Gerber, L.H. (1998). A review of measures of lymphedema. *Cancer Supplement, 83(*12), 2803-2804.

Gould, J., Grassau, P., Manthorne, J., Gray, R. E. & Fitch, M. I. (2006). 'Nothing fit me': nationwide consultations with young women with breast cancer. *Health Expectations, 9,* 158–173.

Gilligan, C. (1982). Visions of maturity. *In a different voice: Psychological theory and women's development.* Cambridge, MA: Harvard University Press.

Giuliano, A.E., Hunt, K.K., Ballman, K.V., Beitsch, P.D., Whitworth, P.W., Blumencranz, P.W., Leitch, A.M., Saha, S., McCall, L.M., Morrow, M. (2011). Axillary dissection vs no axillary dissection in women with invasive breast cancer and sentinel node metastasis: a randomized clinical trial. JAMA: *Journal of American Medical Association, 305*(6):569-575.

Guerin, N., & Dattilo, J. (2001). Family leisure in the context of a chronic disabling condition. *Annual in Therapeutic Recreation, 10,* 73-82, 84-85, 93.

Hamilton, R., Miedema, B., MacIntyre, L., & Easley, J. (2011). Using a positive self-talk intervention to enhance coping skills in breast cancer survivors: lessons from a community-based group delivery model. *Current Oncology, 18*(2), E46-E53.

Heiney, S. P., McWayne, J., Cunningham, J. E., Hazlett, L. J., Parrish, R. S., Bryant, L. H., et al. (2007) Quality of life and lymphedema following breast cancer." *Lymphology,* 40(4), 177-184.

Henderson, K. A., Bialeschki, M.D., Shaw, S. M., & Freysiner, V. J. (1996). *Both gains and gaps: Feminist perspectives on women's leisure.* State College, PA: Venture Publishing.

Henson, H. K. (2002). Breast cancer and sexuality. *Sexuality and Disability, 20*(4), 261-275.

Hill, R. (1949). Families under stress: Adjustment to the crisis of war separation and reunion. New York: Harper and Brothers.

Horner, M. J., Ries, L. A. G., Krapcho, M., et al. (Eds.). (2009). *SEER Cancer Statistics Review, 1975-2006.* National Cancer Institute. Bethesda, MD, http://seer.cancer.gov/csr/1975_2006/, based on November 2008 SEER data submission, posted to the SEER web site, 2009.

Hull, M. M. (1998). Functional and psychosocial aspects of lymphedema in women treated for breast cancer. *Innovations in Breast Cancer Care, 3*(4), 97-100.

Ingoldsby, B.B., Smith, S.R., & Miller, J.E. (2004). *Exploring family theories.* Los Angeles, CA: Roxbury.

International Society of Lymphology [ISL], (2003). The diagnosis and treatment of peripheral lymphedema. *Lymphology, 36,* 84-91.

Jack, D. C. (1991). *Silencing the self: Women and depression.* Cambridge: Harvard University.

Jeruss, J.S., Vicini, F.A., Beitsch, P.D., Haffty, B.G., Quiet, C.A., Zannis, V.J., et al. (2006). Initial outcomes for patients treated on the American Society of Breast Surgeons MammoSite clinical trial for ductal carcinoma-in-situ of the breast. *Annals of Surgical Oncology, 13*(7), 967-976.

Jo, S., Kosciulek, J. F., Huh, C., Holecek, D. F. (2004). Comparison of travel patterns of families with and without a member with a disability. *Journal of Rehabilitation, 70*(4), 34-45.

Johansson, K., Tibe, K., Weibull, A., Newton, R.C. (2005). Low intensity resistance exercise for breast cancer patients with arm lymphedema with or without compression sleeve. *Lymphology, 38*(4):167-180.

Johansson, K., Ohlsson, K., Ingvar, C., Albertsson, M., & Ekdahl, C. (2002). Factors associated with the development of arm lymphedema following breast cancer treatment: A match pair case-control study. *Lymphology, 35*(2), 59-71.

Kedde, H. & van Berlo, W. (2006). Sexual satisfaction and sexual self images of people with physical disabilities in the Netherlands. *Sexuality and Disability, 24* (1), 53-68.

Kim, Y., & Given, B. A. (2008). Quality of life of family caregivers of cancer survivors - Across the trajectory of the illness. *Cancer, 112*(11), 2556-2568.

Koch, P. B., Mandfield, P. K., Thurau, D., & Carey, M. (2005). "Feeling frumpy": The relationships between body image and sexual response changes in midlife women. *The Journal of Sex Research, 42,* 215-223.

Kornblith, A. B., Herndon, J. E., Weiss, R. B., Zhang, C. F., Zuckerman, E. L., Rosenberg, S. M., et al. (2003). Long-term adjustment of survivors of early-stage breast carcinoma, 20 years after adjuvant chemotherapy. *Cancer, 98,* 679–89.

Kosir, M. A., Rymal, C., Koppolu, P., Hryniuk, L., Darga, L., Du, W., et al. (2001). Surgical outcomes after breast cancer surgery: Measuring acute lymphedema. *Journal of Surgical Research, 95*(2), 147-151.

Kwan, W., Jackson, J., Weir, L. M., Dingee, C., McGregor, G., & Olivotto, I. A. (2002). Chronic arm morbidity after curative breast cancer treatment: Prevalence and impact on quality of life. *Journal of Clinical Oncology, 20*(20), 4242-4248.

Lacey, M. (2002). The experience of using decisional support aids by patients with breast cancer. *Oncology Nursing Forum, 29*(10), 1491-1497.

Langer, I., Guller, U., Berclaz, G., Koechli, O.R., Schaer, G., Fehr, M.K., Hess, T., Oertli, D., Bronz, L., Schnarwyler, B., Wight, E., Uehlinger, U., Infanger, E., Burger, D., Zuber, M. (2007). Morbidity of sentinel lymph node biopsy (SLN) alone versus SLN and completion axillary lymph node dissection after breast cancer surgery: a prospective Swiss multicenter study on 659 patients. *Annals of Surgery, 245*(3), 452-61.

Lindau, S. T., Schumm, L. P., Laumann, E. O., Levinson, W., O'Muircheartaigh, C. A., & Waite, L. J. (2007). A study of sexuality and health among older adults in the United States. *The New England Journal of Medicine, 357* (8), 762-774.

Lloyd, C., King, R., Lampe, J., & McDougall, S. (2001). The leisure satisfaction of people with psychiatric disabilities. *Psychiatric Rehabilitation Journal, 25*(2), 107-113.

Loprinzi, C.L., Kugler, J.W., Sloan, J.A., Rooke, T.W., Quella, S.K., Novotny, P., et al. (1999). Lack of effect of coumarin in women with lymphedema after treatment for breast cancer. *New England journal of Medicine, 340,* 346-350.

Mallinger, J., Griggs, J., & Shields, C. (2006). Family communication and mental health after breast cancer. *European Journal of Cancer Care, 15*(4), 355-361.

Mak, S.S., Yeo, W., Lee, Y.M., Mo, K.F., Tse, K.Y., Tse, S.M., Ho, F.P., Kwan., W.H. (2008). Predictors of lymphedema in patients with breast cancer undergoing axillary lymph node dissection in Hong Kong. *Nursing Research, 57*(6), 416- 25.

Maunsell, E., Brisson, J., & Deschenes, L. (1993). Arm problems and psychological distress after surgery for breast cancer. *Canadian Journal of Surgery, 36*(4), 315-320.

Mayrovitz, H.N., Simms, N., & MacDonald, J. (2000). Assessment of limb volume by manual and automated methods in patients with limb edema or lymphedema. *Advances In Skin & Wound Care, 13*(6), 272-276.

McCabe, C., Begley, C., Collier, S., & McCann, S. (2008). Methodological issues related to assessing and measuring quality of life in patients with cancer: implications for patient care. *European Journal of Cancer Care, 17*(1), 56-64.

McCubbin, M. A., & McCubbin, H. I. (1991). Family stress theory and assessment: The resiliency model of family stress, adjustment, and adaptation. In H. I. McCubbin & A. I. Thompson (eds.), Family assessment inventories for research and practice (pp. 3-32). Madison, WI: University of Wisconsin-Madison.

McCubbin, M. A., & McCubbin, H. I. (1996). Resiliency in families: A conceptual model of family adjustment and adaptation in response to stress and crises. In H. I. McCubbin, A. I. Thompson, & M. A. McCubbin (eds.), Family assessment: Resiliency, coping and adaptation-Inventories for research and practice (pp. 1-64). Madison, WI: University of Wisconsin System.

McLaughlin, S. A., Wright, M. J., Morris, K. T., Giron, G. L., Sampson, M. R., Brockway, J. P., et al. (2008). Prevalence of lymphedema in women with breast cancer 5 years after sentinel lymph node biopsy or axillary dissection: objective measurements. *Journal of Clinical Oncology*, 26(32), 5213-5219.

Meek, A.G. (1998). Breast radiotherapy and lymphedema. *Cancer Supplement, 83*(12), 2788-2797.

Megens, A., & Harris, S. (1998). Physical therapist management of lymphedema following treatment for breast cancer: A critical review of its effectiveness. *Physical Therapy, 78*(12), 1302-1311.

Mederer, H. (1993). Division of labor in two-earner homes: Task accomplishment versus household management as critical variables in perceptions about family work. *Journal of Marriage & Family, 55*(1), 133-145.

Mellon, S., & Northouse, L. L. (2001). Family survivorship and quality of life following a cancer diagnosis. *Research in Nursing & Health, 24*, 446-459.

Molassiotis, A. (1997). A conceptual model of adaptation to illness and quality of life for cancer patients treated with bone marrow transplants. *Journal of Advanced Nursing, 26*(3), 572-579.

Mortimer P. (2003). Lymphoedema. In: Warrell DA, Cox TM, Firth JD, eds. Oxford Textbook of Medicine, Vol 2, 2nd ed. Oxford: Oxford University Press:pp.1202–1208.

Mortimer, P.S. (1998). The pathophysiology of lymphedema. *Cancer, 83*(12 Suppl American), 2798-2802.

National Institute on Aging. (2005). AgePage. Sexuality in later life. Gaithersburg, MD: U.S. Department of Health and Human Services.

Northouse, L.L., Laten, D., Reddy, P. (1995). Factors affecting couples' adjustment to recurrent breast cancer. *Social Science & Medicine, 41*(1), 69-76.

O'Brien BM, Mellow CG, Khazanchi RK, et al. (1990). Long-term results after microlymphaticovenous anastomoses for the treatment of obstructive lymphedema. *Plastic Reconstruction Surgery, 85*: 562–72.

Olson, D. H., Lavee, Y. & McCubbin, H. I. (1988). Types of families and family response to stress across the family life cycle. In D. H. Klein & J. Aldous, (eds). *Family stress, coping, and social support* (pp. 48-72). Springfield, IL: Charles C. Thomas.

Olszewski, W. (2000). Clinical efficacy of micronized purified flavonoid fraction (MPFF) in edema. *Angiology, 51*(1):25-29.

Orthner, D. K., & Mancini, J. A. (1990). Leisure impact on family interaction and cohesion. *Journal of Leisure Research, 22*(2), 125-137.

Park, J., Hoffman, L., Marquis, J., Turnbull, A. P., Poston, D., Mannan, H., et al. (2003). Toward assessing family outcomes for service delivery: Validation of a Family Quality of Life Survey. *Journal of Intellectual Disability Research, 47*(5), 367– 384.

Partsch H. (1995). Assessment of abnormal lymph drainage for the diagnosis of lymphedema by isotopic lymphangiography and by indirect lymphography. *Clinical Dermatology, 13*(5):445-450.

Paskett, E.D., Naughton, M.J., McCoy, T.P., Case, L.D., Abbott, J.M. (2007). The epidemiology of arm and hand swelling in premenopausal breast cancer survivors. *Cancer Epidemiology, Biomarkers & Prevention, 16*(4), 75-82.

Passik, S. D., & McDonald, M. V. (1998). Psychosocial aspects of upper extremity lymphedema in women treated for breast carcinoma. *Cancer, 83*(12), 2817-2820.

Passik, S. D., Newman, M., Brennan, M., & Tunkel, R. (1995). Predictors of psychological distress, sexual dysfunction and physical functioning among women with upper extremity lymphedema related to breast cancer. *Psycho-oncology, 4*, 255-263.

Petlund, C.F. (1991). Volumetry of limbs. In W.I. Olszewski (Ed). (1991). *Lymph stasis: Pathophysiology, diagnosis and treatment* (pp. 444-451). Boston: CRC Press.

Petrek, J.A., Senie, R.T., Peters, M., Rosen, P.P. (2001). Lymphedema in a cohort of breast carcinoma survivors 20 years after diagnosis. *Cancer, 92*(6),1368-77.

Pondé, M. P., & Santana, V. S. (2000). Participation in leisure activities: Is it a protective factor for women's mental health? *Journal of Leisure Research, 32*(4), 457-472.

Poston, D., Turnbull, A., Park, J., Mannan, H., Marquis, J., & Wang, M. (2003). Family quality of life: A qualitative inquiry. *Mental Retardation, 41*(5), 313-318.

Pyszel, A., Malyszczak, K., Pyszel, K., Andrzejak, R., Szuba, A. (2006). Disability, psychological distress and quality of life in breast cancer survivors with arm lymphedema. *Lymphology, 39*(4),185-92.

Radina, M. E. (2009). Breast cancer-related lymphedema: Implications for family leisure participation. *Family Relations, 58*(4), 445-459.

Radina, M. E., & Armer, J. M. (2001). Post breast cancer lymphedema and the family: A qualitative investigation of families coping with chronic illness. *Journal of Family Nursing, 7*, 281-299.

Radina, M. E., & Armer, J. M. (2004). Surviving breast cancer and living with lymphedema: Resiliency among women in the context of their families. *Journal of Family Nursing, 10*(4), 485-505.

Radina, M. E., Armer, J. M., & Stewart, B. (under review). Making self-care a priority for women at-risk for breast cancer- related lymphedema. *Journal of Family Psychology.*

Radina, M. E., Watson, W. K., & Faubert, K. (2009). Breast cancer-related lymphoedema and sexual relationships in mid and later life. *Journal of Lymphoedema, 3(2), 20-37.*

Raveis, V.H., & Pretter, S. (2004). Existential plight of adult daughters following their mother's breast cancer diagnosis. *Psycho-Oncology,* 14, 49-60.

Rees, C. E., & Bath, P. A. (2000). The information needs and source preferences of women with breast cancer and their family members: A review of the literature published between 1988 and 1998. *Journal of Advanced Nursing, 31*(4), 833-841.

Rettig, K. D., & Leichtentritt, R. D. (1999). A general theory for perceptual indicators of family life quality. *Social Indicators Research, 47*, 307-342.

Ridner, S. H. (2002). Breast cancer lymphedema: Pathophysiology and risk reduction guidelines. *Oncology Nursing Forum, 29*(9), 1285-1293.

Ridner, S.H. (2005). Quality of life and a symptom cluster associated with breast cancer treatment-related lymphedema. *Supportive Care in Cancer, 13,* 904-911.

Ridner, S.H. (2006). Pretreatment lymphedema education and identified educational resources in breast cancer patients. *Patient Education & Counseling, 61*(1), 72-79.

Ridner, S. H., Dietrich, M. S., & Kidd, N. (2011). Breast cancer treatment-related lymphedema self-care: Education, practices, symptoms, and quality of life. *Supportive Care in Cancer, 19*, 631-637.

Ridner, S., Montgomery, L., Hepworth, J., Stewart, B.R., & Armer, J. (2007). Comparison of upper limb volume measurement techniques and arm symptoms between healthy volunteers and individuals with known lymphedema. *Lymphology, 40*, 35-46.

Ridner, S.H., Murphy, B., Deng, J., Kidd, N., Galford, E., Dietrich, M.S. (2010). Advanced pneumatic therapy in self-care of chronic lymphedema of the trunk. *Lymphatic Research & Biology, 8*(4):209-15.

Rinehart-Ayres, M.E. (1998). Conservative approaches to lymphedema treatment. *Cancer, 83*(12 Suppl American), 2828-2832.

Rockson, S.G. (1998). Precipitating factors in lymphedema: Myths and realities. *Cancer Supplement, 83*(12), 2814-2816.

Rockson, S.G., Miller, L.T., & Senie, R. (1998). Workgroup III. Diagnosis and management of lymphedema. *Cancer Supplement, 83*(12), 2882-2885.

Ruddick, S. (1989). Maternal thinking as a feminist standpoint. *Maternal thinking: Toward a politics of peace,* (p. 127-139). Boston: Beacon Press.

Schmitz KH, Troxel AB, Cheville A, et al. Physical activity and lymphedema (the PAL trial): Assessing the safety of progressive strength training in breast cancer survivors. *Contemp Clin Trials.* May 2009;30(3):233-245.

Smith-Bird, E., & Turnbull, A. P. (2005). Linking positive behavior support to family quality-of-life outcomes. *Journal of Positive Behaviors Interventions, 7*(3), 174-180.

Stanton, A.W., Modi, S., Mellor, R.H., Levick, J.R., & Mortimer, P.S. (2009).Recent advances in breast cancer-related lymphedema of the arm: lymphatic pump failure and predisposing factors. *Lymphatic Research & Biology, 7*(1):29-45.

Stanton, A.W.B., Northfield, J.W., Holroyd, P.S., Mortimer, P.S., & Levick, J.R. (1997). Validation of an optoelectronic limb volumeter (Perometer). *Lymphology, 30*, 77-79.

Stout Gergich, N.L., Pfalzer, L.A., McGarvey, C., Springer, B., Gerber L.H., Soballe, P. (2008). Preoperative assessment enables the early diagnosis and successful treatment of lymphedema. *Cancer, 112*(12), 2809-19.

Taleporos, G., Dip, G., & McCabe, M. P. (2002). The impact of sexual esteem, body esteem, and sexual satisfaction on psychological well-being in people with physical disability. *Sexuality and Disability, 20* (3), 177-183.

Ter, S.E., Alavi, A., Kim, C.K., Merli, G. (1993). Lymphoscintigraphy. A reliable test for the diagnosis of lymphedema. *Clinical Nuclear Medicine, 18*(8):646-654.

Thiadens, S.R.J. (1998). Current status of education and treatment resources for lymphedema. *Cancer Supplement, 83*(12), 2864-2868.

Thomas-MacLean, R., Miedema, B., & Tatemichi, S. R. (2005). Breast cancer-related lymphedema: Women's experiences with an underestimated condition. *Canadian Family Physician, 51*, 246-247.

Tierney, S., Aslam, M., Rennie, K., & Grace, P. (1996). Infrared optoelectronic volumetry, the ideal way to measure limb volume. *European Journal of Vascular and Endovascular Surgery, 12*(4), 412-417.

Vaidya, J.S., Baum, M., Tobias, J.S., Massarut, S., Wenz, F., Murphy. O., et al. (2006). Targeted intraoperative radiotherapy (TARGIT) yields very low recurrence rates when given as a boost. *International Journal of Radiation Oncology, Biology, Physics, 66*(5), 1335-1338.

Vassard, D., Olsen, M. H., Zinckernagel, L., Vibe-Petersen, J., Dalton, S. O., & Johansen, J. (2010). Psychological consequences of lymphoedema associated with breast cancer: A prospective cohort study." *European Journal of Cancer, 46*(18), 3211-3218.

Voogd, A. C., Ververs, J. M., Vingerhoets, A. J., Roumen, R. M., Coebergh, J. W., & Crommelin, M. A. (2003). Lymphoedema and reduced shoulder function as indicators of quality of life after axillary lymph node dissection for invasive breast cancer. *British Journal of Surgery, 90*(1), 76-81.

Ward, L.C., Bunce, I.H., Cornish, B.H., Mirolo, B.R., Thomas, B.J., & Jones, L.C. (1992). Multi-frequency bioelectrical impediance augments the diagnosis and management of lymphoedema in post-mastectomy patients. *European Journal of Clinical Invesigation, 22*(11), 751-754.

Ward, L.C., Essex, T., & Cornish, B.H., (2006). Determination of Cole parameters in multiple frequency bioelectrical impedance analysis using only the measurement of impedances. *Physiological Measurement, 27*(9), 839-850.

Wiederman, M. W. & Hurst, S. R. (1997). Physical attractiveness, body image, and women's sexual self-schema. *Psychology of Women Quarterly, 21*, 567-580.

Zabriskie, R. (2000). *An examination of family and leisure behaviors among families with middle school aged children*. Unpublished dissertation. Indiana University, Bloomington, IN.

Zabriskie, R., & McCormick, B. (2001). The influences of family leisure patterns on perceptions of family functioning. *Family Relations, 50*(3), 66-74.

Zabriskie, R., & McCormick, B. (2003). Parent and child perspectives of family leisure involvement and satisfaction with family life. *Journal of Leisure Research, 35*(2), 163-189.

5

Pelvic Lymphedema in Rectal Cancer

Alberto Vannelli and Luigi Battaglia
Fondazione IRCCS "Istituto Nazionale dei Tumori", Milan, Italy

1. Introduction

Clarke's Second Law is: "The only way of discovering the limits of the possible is to venture a little way past them into the impossible" (Clarke, 1962). Pelvic lymphedema issues this challenge.

The prognosis for pelvic malignancies has improved in recent years mainly due to advanced technologies and better knowledge of the pathways of cancer spread. Lymphadenectomy is the most important prognostic factor in pelvic malignancies, a finding that has substantially changed surgical approaches from a "quantitative" premise to a more "qualitative" nature giving priority to the psycho-physical integrity of cancer patients by limiting the surgical intervention (Breyer et al, 2008; Mills et al, 2006; Desnoo & Faithfull 2006; Greco et al, 2006).

However, despite progress made by the conservative surgical approach for rectal cancer, the development of functional abnormalities in patients undergoing conservative surgery has become more evident (Ortiz & Armendariz, 1996). These dysfunctional pathology are associated with symptoms similar to those of the pre-surgery pelvic pathology. Most importantly these problems are considered a major public health issue representing one third of costs of colorectal cancer treatment, even if the massive economic burden of disability has received limited attention (Selke, 2003). Although theories including neural damage, reduction of capacity and compliance of organs, and sensory loss have been already proposed, no clear evidence of a direct correlation between such symptoms and surgical damage exists. Additionally, such disabilities do not depend on the extent of the surgical intervention (conservative versus radical), on the use of concomitant post-operative radio-chemotherapy or the gender (Kakodkar et al, 2006). Fortunately, patients have been shown to respond to biofeedback reeducation of the pelvic floor, with or without added psychotherapy (Devroede, 1999).

We hypotized that pelvic surgery, regardless of the extra-peritoneal organs, results in the loss of continuity of the pelvic region, as key event with the following reduction in fatty tissue where the lymph node stations are mostly concentrated. Therefore we suggest that pelvic lymphadenectomy should be followed by a pelvic lymphedema (Vannelli et al, 2009).

Once identified, lymphedema does not undergo significant reabsorption and may lead to serious chronic pathology with severe functional impairment of pelvic organs ((Zermann et al, 2001). Yet, the mechanisms and pathways that involve lymphedema in pelvic pathology are still unknown and needs to be investigated. We examined, by chance, post surgery lymphedema in 13 patients submitted to our hospital for colorectal adenocarcinoma, by comparing MRI of the abdominal area of the pre and post surgery. Interestingly, comparison of dynamic MRI images obtained in different phases of the patient's management enabled identification of pelvic floor lymphedema after surgical intervention for colorectal adenocarcinoma.

2. Vannelli's theory

The complete description of the lymphatic vessels goes back to 17th century. However, some investigators have only recently recognized the impact of lymphology on the treatment of tumours, both from research and clinical points of view. This sudden increased interest has led to study oncological and functional lymphatic disease, in particular related to lymphedema. It is known that each lymphadenectomy is associated to a lymphedema. Lymphedema is defined as a chronic and debilitating condition and it is correct to suggest the presence of a lymphedema also in the pelvic area related to the oncological surgery treatment: a pelvic lymphedema, that we will call blind lymphedema, i.e. with symptoms but with no signs. We make an introduction. Are we sure to know the meaning of lymphedema? Lymphedema is what we know because we can see it: upper limbs, lower limbs, even neck, scrotum or pubis (Thorat, 2006; Fang et al, 2008; Vignes & Trévidic, 2005). Probably there is a lymphedema that we do not know only because we cannot see it. The Roman playwright Terentius wrote: ''But 'even if the old masters have discovered everything, one thing will be always new, - the application and the scientific study and classification of the discoveries made by others. " (Gummere, 1917-28). To clear our mind of any doubt, it is necessary to make a step backwards. In the scientific discussion lymphedema is not a ''meaning" that does not define or indicate a disorder. It is rather defined by its characteristics, i.e. what determines a lymphedema: interstitial retention of proteins, tissue inflammation, fatty tissue hypertrophy, fibrosis, progressive pathological condition, but this is not lymphedema (Warren et al, 2007). The only acceptable definition of lymphedema should be the alteration of the lymphatic vessels due to a (primary) malformation or a (secondary) mechanical damage. Basing on this definition, a new model of lymphedema can be therefore assumed: pelvic lymphedema, that is the alteration of lymphatic vessels associated to a pelvis mechanical damage. The pelvic disorders are extremely frequently and occur regardless of gender, type of surgery or concomitant medical treatment (pre- or post-operative radiotherapy). The study on pelvic disorders immediately is found to be of difficult execution and even without instrumental evidence of any damage, an important symptomatology can be present. The available examinations for the study of the various pelvic components are numerous: uroflowmetry and cystography to investigate the bladder; rectomanometry or electrical stimulation by means of evoked potentials of pudendal nerve; defecography for the investigation of the rectum, just to mention some of them. However, the available data in the literature do not give any satisfactory response concerning the patients with negative tests but with clinically relevant disorders (Antolak et al, 2002). Perineology has acquired higher importance in the recent years: a multispecialistic discipline of multifactorial interest of pelvic diseases with rehabilitation purpose (Peters et al, 2008). After a careful follow-up of the patients operated for pelvic tumours, we observed that all the patients referring to the perineology centres had a relevant benefit from the rehabilitation treatment reducing the complications rate and, in some cases, preventing them (Bai et al, 2006; Brown & Seow-Choen, 2000). This could answer the question "how does pelvic lymphedema occur?" During surgery the main responsible of the damage should be detected because if, not promptly treated, it can result in a chronic disease. However, to promptly institute the most suitable therapy, we should understand "why does the lymphedema occurs?" and identify the first action. When we talk about postoperative disorders of pelvic surgery, two areas are identified: perineum and extraperitoneal region (Corton, 2005). Perineum consists of soft tissues which close the lower pelvic cavity. This region is sited between the upper portions of the two thighs, to which anal canal, extraperitoneal rectum and external genitals are connected. An ideal transversal line joining the two ischiatic eminences divides the region into two triangles: one anterior, or urogenital perineum, and the other, posterior or anorectal perineum. The subcutaneous layer is bulky in the side walls and posteriorly where it continues with the fat of the ischiorectal fossae.

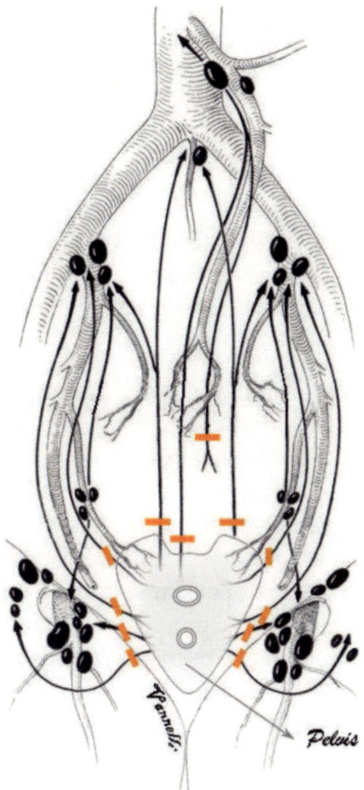

Fig. 1. Illustration of the drainage pathways of the lymphatic vessels in the pelvic area (orange lines correspond to lymphadenectomy and eventfully lymphatic spread).

This allows the proliferation of a rich and branched lymphatic net with numerous lymph nodal stations. The extraperitoneal pelvic space is sited between the peritoneum covering the pelvic organs, and the pelvic diaphragm. In the pelvic cavity the peritoneum is separated from the walls which delimit the cavity by the surrounding and supporting fatty extraperitoneal tissue. This creates a sort of floating effect of the organs contained in the pelvis. The fatty tissue forms the two thirds of the total volume and contains important lymph node stations. The pelvic floor can be considered as the centre supporting the perineal layer. It consists of a complex of muscles which are twisted together and close the pelvis in the bottom.

These muscles wrap the urinary (urethra and bladder) and reproductive (vagina in females and prostate in men) systems and form the anterior floor down to the anorectal apparatus (anus, rectum) which makes the posterior floor. Perineum is a dynamic organ and is continuously subject to our body weight. It especially has the duty to support the increases in intra-abdominal pressure due to the increases in loads, chronic conditions and natural events, such as the childbirth (Van der Putte, 2005). Pelvic surgery, regardless of the involved organs, results in the loss of continuity of the pelvic region as key event with the following reduction in fatty tissue where the lymph node stations are mostly concentrated (Andrade & Jacomo, 2007). Therefore, the occurrence of pelvic disorders, even though of difficult etiology, could be possible due to a surgery which is associated to a lymphadenectomy (Fig. 1). The presence of a lymphadenectomy, that can be considerably wide in some cases, should be followed by a lymphedema.

3. Materials and methods

3.1 Patients

Between March 1990 and January 2010, 6975 patients were operated for colo-rectal carcinoma in the Division of Colorectal Surgery at the Fondazione IRCCS "Istituto Nazionale dei Tumori", a non university teaching hospital in Milan, the Italy.

For the purpose of the study, information was collected both from medical records and a computerized database of patients admitted to our Division, between May 2008 and January 2010. To discriminate pelvic lymphedema we compared the extra-peritoneal adenocarcinoma (cases) with intra-peritoneal adenocarcinoma (controls) staging with MRI examination. Excluded from the analysis were patients with preoperative treatment, those patients with locoregional recurrence, previous pelvic surgery or patients with distant metastases and with more than one primary cancer. We regarded the rectum cut-off within 15 cm from the anal verge and intraperitoneal cut-off more than 12 cm from the anal verge. We identified a cohort of 13 patients with sigmoid colon and rectal adenocarcinoma. Bowel preparation and surgical techniques have been described in details (Leo et al, 2009). All patients had a pre-operative (one week before surgery) and post-operative (six months following discharge from the hospital) MRI examination. This study was approved by the institutional review board.

3.2 Nuclear magnetic resonance

In details, a 1.5-T high-resolution MRI system (Avanto; Siemens Medical Systems, Erlangen, Germany) was used for the pre operative stages and the follow-up of the patients. For the purpose of our study, the 13 patients were examined in the supine position with feet forward and measurements were obtained using the same system and by the same technician.

We consider the common features of lymphedema, usually observed in an MRI examination: circumferential edema, increased volume of subcutaneous tissue, and a honeycomb pattern above the fascia between muscle and subcutaneous fat, with evident thickening of the dermis (Witte, 2002). Although it is generally difficult to differentiate primary from secondary lymphedema, MRI is able to discriminate lymphedema from lipoedema and phlebedema (Lohrmann et al, 2009; Aström et al, 2001). Our standard procedure for pre-operative patients is an MRI with Gadolinium. On the other hand, for follow-ups, the MRI is indicated only for a suspicious local recurrence. Thirteen patients were selected for our study to be evaluated with MRI but with a different approach. In details, along with the above described standard procedures, a sequence of fat-suppressed T2-weighted (FST2) and diffusion weighted T2-weighted (DIT2) were performed, as those are the most efficient techniques to evaluate lymphedema. Specifically, to evaluate lymphedema using FST2 the signal should be increase as the presence of increasing degrees of edema related to active inflammation (Delfaut et al, 1999). Additionally, DIT2 has been found to improve the detection of edema and herein introduced to detect the lymphedema degree (Ebisu T, et al 1993). Moreover when lipoedema occurs, MRI is able to confirm that the peripheral lymphatic system is normal while soft tissue swelling consists solely of fat, and subcutaneous edema is absent.

4. Result

At the time of the analyses thirteen patients were admitted to our department, for colo-rectal adenocarcinoma. Five were male and eight females with a median age of 66, ranging from 45 to 72 years. In all patients, a whole body mass index (BMI) was calculated: range 25-35, mean 29.9. Cases included patients with adenocarcinoma of the sigmoid colon without metastases and rectum without metastases. Four patients have been affected by intra-peritoneal adenocarcinoma: one sigmoid and three upper third rectal cancer (one male and three female) and nine extra-peritoneal adenocarcinoma: four middle third rectal cancer and five lower third rectal cancer (four male and five female). The patients affected by intra-peritoneal adenocarcinoma has been submitted to: one resection of sigmoid colon and three anterior resection of upper rectum. Three patient presented stage IIa and one stage I. The patients affected by extra-peritoneal adenocarcinoma has been submitted to seven anterior resection of the rectum and two total resection of the rectum with colo-endo anal anastomosis. Seven patient presented stage I and two stage 0. Nine patients with an extra-peritoneal lesion underwent a resection of middle and lower third of rectum with regional lymphadenectomy, while the other patients with an intra-peritoneal lesion required resection of sigmoid colon and upper third of the rectum with regional lymphadenectomy. A sagittal and coronal T1 MRI, as well as FST2 and DIT2 images on the axial plane were requested for the seven patients who underwent anterior rectal resection, which involved the pelvic floor, as a result of extra-peritoneal location of the adenocarcinoma (middle and lower third of the rectum). There is no clear evidence of the pelvic lymphedema or lymphatic alterations in the pre-operative MRI performed 1 week prior to surgery for all patients. However, a post-operative MRI follow-up performed six months flowing discharge from the hospital revealed in seven patients a lymphatic 'stipes-like' elements within the presacral adipose tissue with compression of the sacro-sciatic ligaments and bladder, all indicative of lymphatic alterations. Moreover in nine patients, the area of edema and venous congestion of pelvis together with compression of pelvic organs indicated by MRI signals, were located far from the area of surgical intervention. Furthermore, in eight patients, with the phase of T1 acquisition, epifascial "lakes" related to the muscular bands located outside of the pelvic floor in gluteal muscles were identified. Additionally, in six patients, the DIT2 enabled the detection of moderate lymphatic stasis in the presacral space. On the other hand, the four patients who underwent resection of the sigmoid colon and upper third of the rectum (without pelvic involvement due to intra-peritoneal adenocarcinoma located more than 12 cm from the anal verge), had a different MRI outcome. In details, the axial second planes were amplified with acquisition of T1, FST2 and DIT2- weighted sagittal and coronal images through subtraction of adipose tissue signals on the axial planes. Pre-operative MRI revealed no pelvic lymphedema or alterations of the pelvic lymphatics in these patients. Also the post-operative follow-up performed six months after discharge from the hospital, showed no evidence of pelvic wall edema. Two patients, submitted to resection of the sigmoid colon, presented mild signal intensification in the lower part of the rectal abdominal muscle (figure 6). Overall, there are no signs of lymphatic congestion anywhere within the pelvic wall were noted in the four patients with intra-peritoneal surgery. Table I summarizes surgery information for each patient. Thirteen patients were admitted to our department for colo-rectal adenocarcinoma. Five were males and 8 females with a median age of 66, ranging from 45 to 72 years. In all patients, a whole body mass index (BMI) was calculated: range 25-35, mean 29.9.

Number patient	Age	Sex	Body Mass Index	Site of cancer	Surgical procedure	Cancer classification
1	45	female	25	Sigmoid colon	RSC	IIa
2	72	male	35	URC	ARR	IIa
3	68	female	31,6	URC	ARR	IIa
4	70	female	25,8	URC	ARR	I
5	55	female	29,9	URC	ARR	I
6	60	male	28,8	MRC	ARR	I
7	59	female	29,6	LRC	ARR	0
8	71	female	29,9	LRC	ARR	I
9	66	male	28,9	MRC	ARR	I
10	65	female	31,2	MRC	CEAA	0
11	64	female	33,5	LRC	ARR	I
12	67	male	34,5	LRC	CEEA	I
13	67	male	33,3	LRC	ARR	I

Upper third rectal cancer (URC), Middle third rectal cancer (MRC), Low third rectal cancer (LRC), Resection of the sigmoid colon (RSC), Anterior resection of the rectum (ARR), Total resection of the rectum with colo-endo anal anastomosis (CEAA); Cancer classification with American Joint Committee on Cancer Staging 2010

Table 1. Characteristics of patients from May 2008 to January 2010

Cases included patients with adenocarcinoma of the sigmoid colon without metastases and of the rectum without metastases. Four patients have been affected by intra-peritoneal adenocarcinoma: one sigmoid and 3 upper third rectal cancer (1 male and 3 female) and 9 extra-peritoneal adenocarcinoma: 4 middle third rectal cancer and 5 lower third rectal cancer (4 male and 5 female). The patients affected by intra-peritoneal adenocarcinoma have been submitted to: one resection of sigmoid colon and 3 anterior resection of upper rectum. Specifically, 3 patients presented stage IIa and one stage I. The patients affected by extra-peritoneal adenocarcinoma have been submitted to 7 anterior resection of the rectum and 2 total resection of the rectum with colo-endo anal anastomosis. In details, 7 patients presented stage I, and 2 stage 0. Nine patients with an extra-peritoneal lesion underwent a resection of middle and lower third of rectum with regional lymphadenectomy, while the other patients with an intra-peritoneal lesion required resection of sigmoid colon and upper third of the rectum with regional lymphadenectomy. Table II summarizes the MRI characteristics for each patient using 4 paramenters: stipes-like, edema and venous congestion, epifascial 'lakes', lymphatic stasis in presacral space.

Patient	Stipes like		Edema and venous congestion		Epifascial "lakes"		Lymphatic stasis in presacral space	
	MRI pre	MRI post	MRI pre	MRI post	MRI pre	MRI post	MRI pre	MRI post
1	no	no	no	no	no	no	no	no
2	no	no	no	no	no	no	no	no
3	no	no	no	no	no	no	no	no
4	no	no	no	no	no	no	no	no
5	no	yes	no	yes	no	yes	no	yes
6	no	no	no	yes	no	yes	no	yes
7	no	no	no	yes	no	yes	no	no
8	no	yes	no	yes	no	no	no	no
9	no	yes	no	yes	no	yes	no	yes
10	no	yes	no	yes	no	yes	no	no
11	no	yes	no	yes	no	yes	no	yes
12	no	yes	no	yes	no	yes	no	yes
13	no	yes	no	yes	no	yes	no	yes

Table 2. MRI characteristics

A sagittal and coronal T1 MRI, as well as FST2 and DIT2 images on the axial plane were requested for the 7 patients who underwent anterior rectal resection, which involved the pelvic floor, as a result of extra-peritoneal location of the adenocarcinoma (middle and lower third of the rectum). There is no clear evidence of the pelvic lymphedema or lymphatic alterations in the pre-operative MRI performed 1 week prior to surgery for all patients (figure 2).

However, a post-operative MRI follow-up performed 6 months flowing discharge from the hospital revealed in 7 patients a lymphatic 'stipes-like' elements within the presacral adipose tissue with compression of the sacro-sciatic ligaments and bladder, all indicative of lymphatic alterations (figure 3). Moreover in 9 patients, the area of edema and venous congestion of pelvis together with compression of pelvic organs indicated by MRI signals, were located far from the area of surgical intervention (figure 4). Furthermore, in 8 patients, with the phase of T1 acquisition, epifascial "lakes" related to the muscular bands located outside of the pelvic floor in gluteal muscles were identified (figure 5). Additionally, in 6 patients, the DIT2 enabled the detection of moderate lymphatic stasis in the presacral space (figure 6). On the other hand, the 4 patients who underwent resection of the sigmoid colon and upper third of the rectum (without pelvic involvement due to intra-peritoneal adenocarcinoma located more than 12 cm from the anal verge), had a different MRI outcome. In details, the axial second planes were amplified with acquisition of T1, FST2 and DIT2- weighted sagittal and coronal images through subtraction of adipose tissue signals on the axial planes. Pre-operative MRI revealed no pelvic lymphedema or alterations of the pelvic lymphatics in these patients. Also the post-operative follow-up performed six months after discharge from the hospital, showed no evidence of pelvic wall edema. Two patients (number 1 and 4), submitted to resection of the sigmoid colon, presented mild signal intensification in the lower part of the rectal abdominal muscle (figure 7). Overall, there are no signs of lymphatic congestion anywhere within the pelvic wall were noted in the four patients with intra-peritoneal surgery.

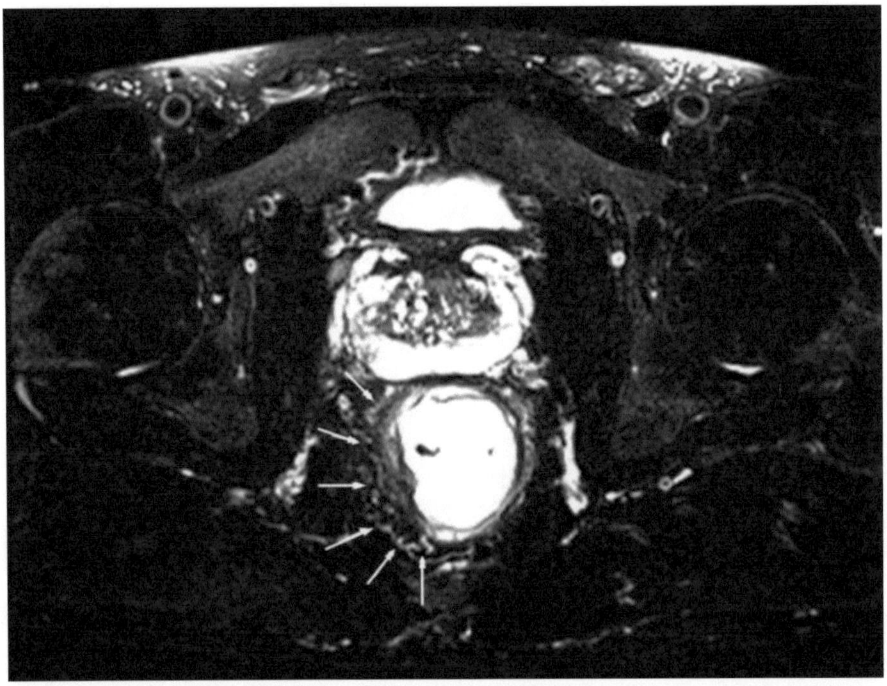

Fig. 2. Phase of FST2 acquisition in pre-operative period, revealing no evidence of lymphedema. Arrows indicate the primary lesion.

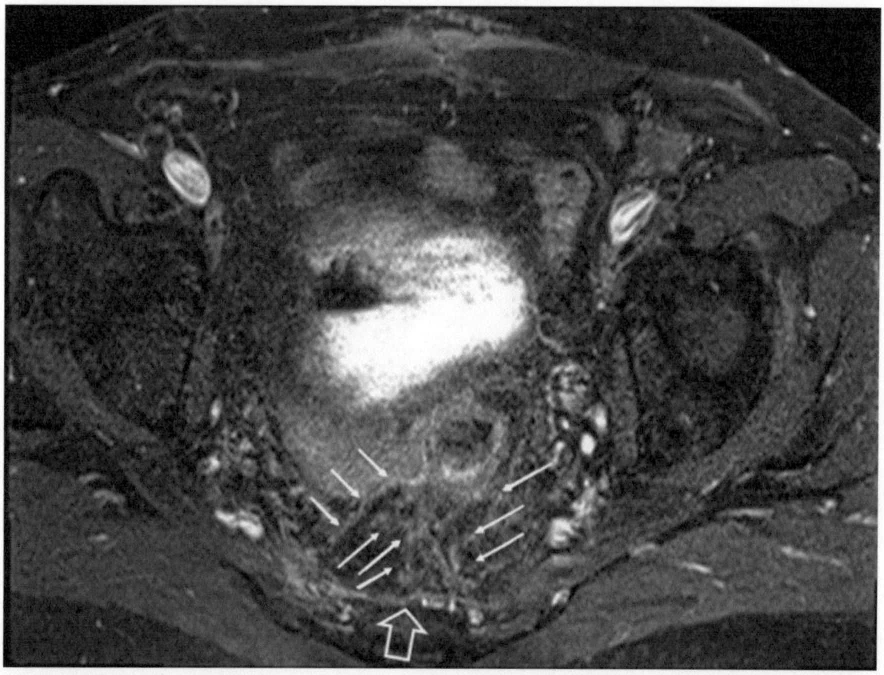

Fig. 3. Post-operative period. Phase of FST2 acquisition. White arrows indicate lymphangitis in the sacral area; large open arrow indicates presacral fibrosis.

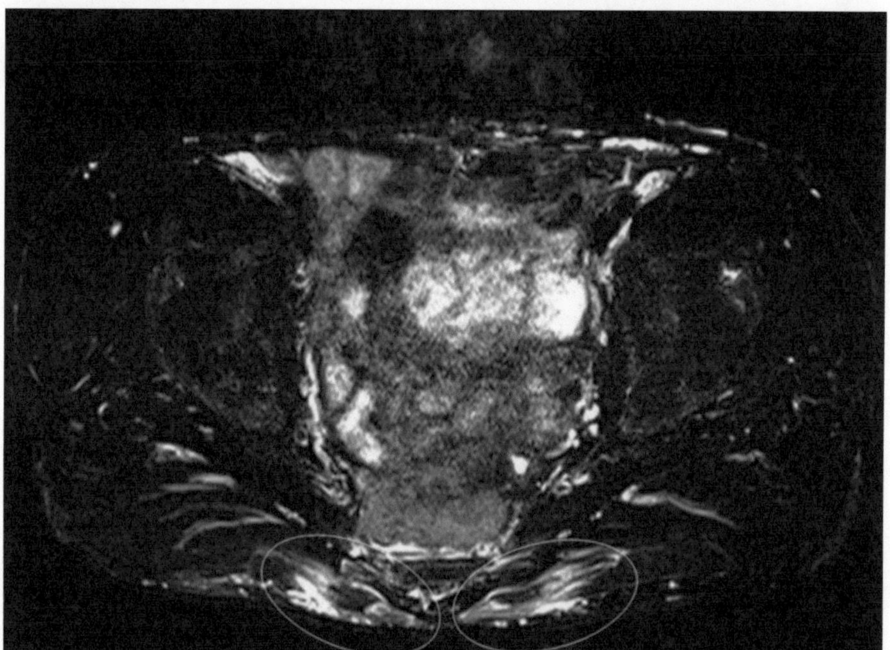

Fig. 4. Post-operative period. Phase of FST2 acquisition. Note lymphedema and venous congestion in presacral area.

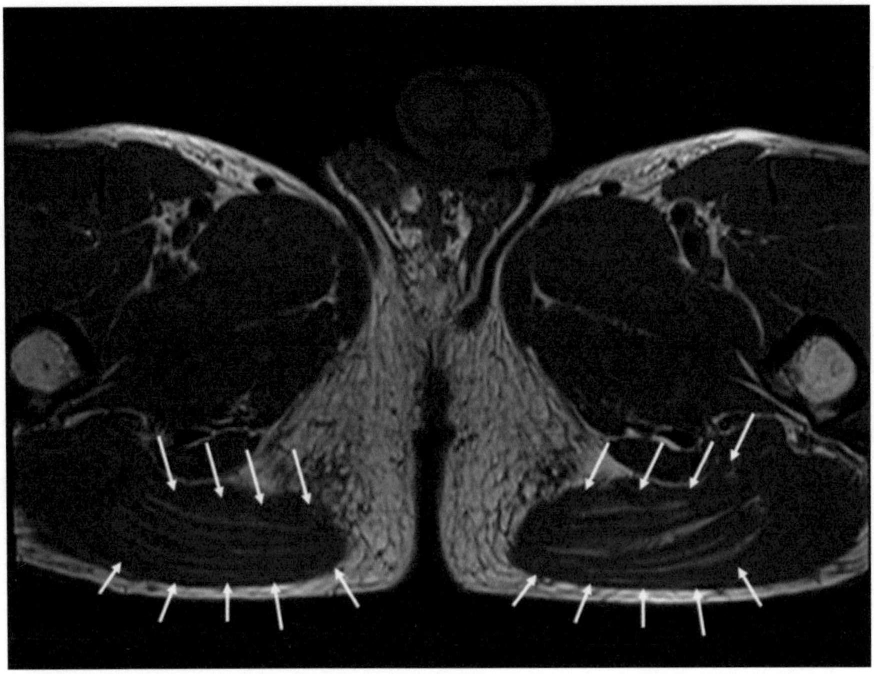

Fig. 5. Post-operative period. Phase of T1 acquisition. Arrows surrounding muscular fascia indicate the epifascial "lakes".

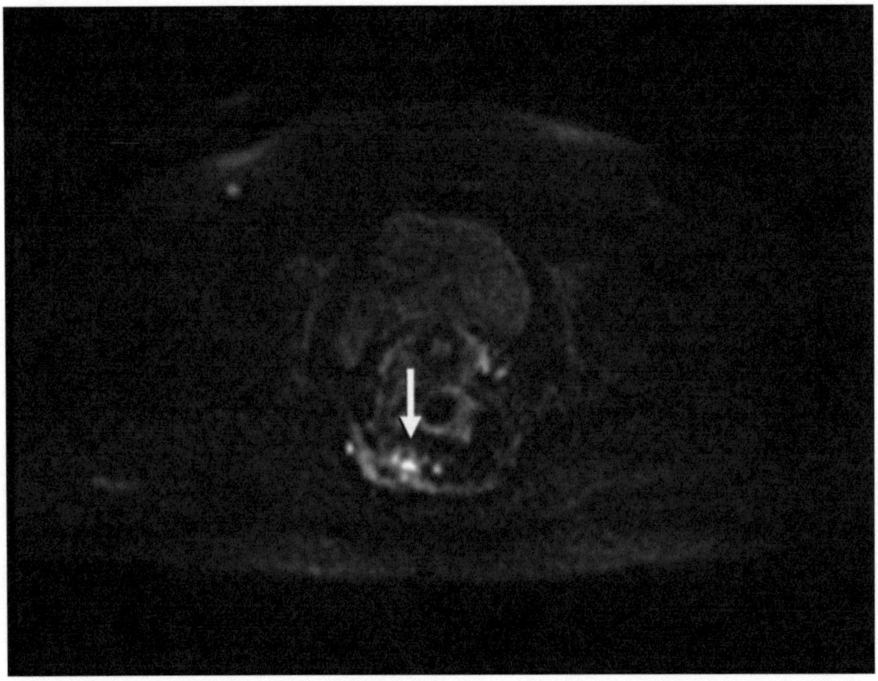

Fig. 6. Post-operative period. Phase of T2WI. Arrow indicates lymphedema in the presacral space.

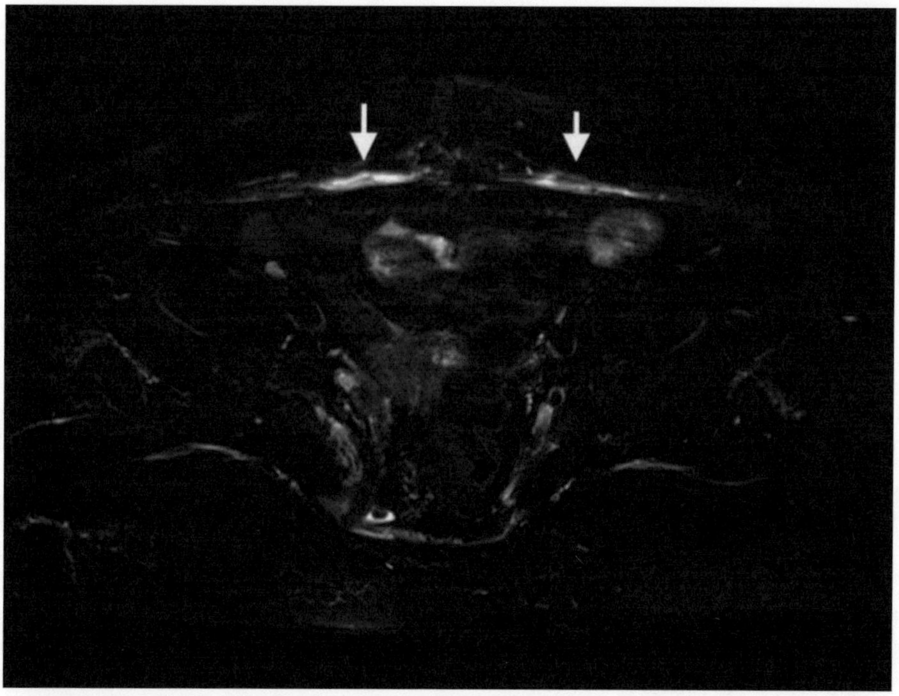

Fig. 7. Post-operative period. Phase of FST2 acquisition. Arrows indicate mild hyperintensity in the area of abdominal rectal muscles.

5. Discussion

5.1 Pathophysiology of the pelvis

Pelvic cavity is a large region. The pelvic bone walls are completed with layered muscles: internal by pyriform and obturators, and closed in the bottom by levator ani and ischiococcygeal muscles which form the pelvic diaphragm or floor. In the pelvic cavity, like in the remaining abdominal cavity, peritoneum is separated from the walls which delimit the cavity by the extraperitoneal connective tissue. Peritoneum surrounds the organs contained in the pelvis is connected backwards with the extraperitoneal tissue, anteriorly with the connective tissue of the anterior compartment of the thigh through the obturator canals, laterally with that of the gluteal regions through the supra- and sub-pyriform canals of the great ischiatic foramen. The extraperitoneal connective tissue occupies the spaces free of viscera. In some points, such as around the rectum and bladder, it looks like a loose fatty connective tissue, while in others it gets thicker and forms septa and ligaments. These are, sometimes, provided with small bundles of smooth muscle cells which have the duty to support the pelvic viscera. These septa are the weak points of the whole pelvis. The septa, that can be hardly delimited from the adjacent loose tissue, surround the vessels directed to viscera or pelvic walls and are rich in lymphatic vessels and lymph nodes too (Wilting et al, 2004). It is, therefore, evident that any surgery in this area should be necessarily associated to a loss of potentially vital substance to perform a really radical lymphoadenectomy. The female pelvic cavity has a different aspect from the male cavity due to the particular development of the genital apparatus. While the male genital apparatus is hidden by the bladder, in the female uterus and its appendages acquire a considerable development: they rise from the extraperitoneal areal tissue and raise the serosa forming ligaments.

Uterus and ligaments, therefore, form a transversal septum which divides the pelvic cavity into an anterior portion, where bladder is sited, and a posterior one occupied by the rectum. Some lymphatic vessels of the rectal ampulla join at the root of the superior rectal vein to reach the anorectal and superior sacral lymph nodes, while others go up to the hypogastric lymph nodes. The bladder lymphatic vessels mouth into the hypogastric and external iliac lymph nodes.

In males the lymphatic vessels of the deferent canal and seminal vesicles are confluents of the external and internal iliac lymph nodes.

The prostate lymphatic vessels mouth into the hypogastric ones, while those of the anterior face of the prostate are confluents of anterior vesical lymph nodes or obturator lymph nodes. Regarding females, the lymphatic vessels of uterus are the following: the fundus uteri lymphatic vessels follow the ovarian vessels and are confluents to lumboaortic lymph nodes sited at the level of the renal hilus; some of the corpus and fundus uteri follow the round ligaments and reach inguinal lymph nodes, whereas those of the corpus and neck reach the internal iliac lymph nodes like those of vagina. In the pelvic extraperitoneal region lymphatic vessels follow the course of parietal and visceral veins and present lymph nodes alternating along their course.

Those distributed along the internal iliac vessels that receive lymphatic collectors of pelvic viscera and walls are particularly relevant. Finally, the pelvic cavity is externally closed by the perineum which is made by a diamond-shaped layer rich in fatty tissue. The most superficial lymphatic vessels are confluents of inguinal lymph nodes, while the internal ones go along the blood vessels and anastomose with the anal ones. The perineum in the posterior portion is crossed by anus whose lymphatic vessels which come from the columnar area and haemorrhoidal ring are confluents of internal iliac lymph nodes. The vessels of the anal orifice are confluents of the anorectal lymph nodes and inguinal lymph nodes of the medial group. The perineum in the anterior portion has a similar structure in both genders.

The constituting layers are, however, modified by the different conformation of the genital organs. In male two lymphatic pathways for the penis can be identified. The first consisting of superficial lymphatic vessels which join together in a unique trunk which flows with the dorsal superficial vein and mouths into the superficial inguinal lymph nodes and then bifurcates together with those coming from the scrotum. The second is constituted by deep lymphatic vessels which join in an unpaired dorsal trunk which goes with the anonymous vein and join the external iliac lymph nodes. The lymphatic vessels of testicle follow the spermatic cord and flow into lumboaortic lymph nodes. In the female, the lymphatic vessels of the mons of pubis, labia majora and minora are confluents of superficial inguinal lymph nodes. The lymphatic vessels of erectile organs are confluents of deep inguinal lymph nodes or external iliac vessels. It is evident how the pathways of lymphatic outflow of pelvis are extremely branched and the lymph node stations constitute a closely inter-connected complex.

Moreover, contrary to the remaining areas, these lymphatic pathways are exposed to a high pressure for two reasons: to counteract the pressure difference between endo-abdominal and endo-thoracic values and due to the calibre of the outflow vessels, which are particularly large (cisterna of Pecquet, lumbar right and left lymphatic trunks). The oncological surgery in the pelvic area always involves a remarkable radical operation of lymph nodes, which is partially necessary (lymphoadenectomy), but also unavoidable. The removal of extraperitoneal tissue occupying the areas free from viscera is, as mentioned above, abundantly supplied by lymphatic vessels. The lymphatic pathway on the transected area is completed removed without having any alternative outflow pathways (Taneja & Cady, 2005). It is appropriate to assume that the lymphedema related to lymphoadenectomy appears in the same way as it occurs in other body areas. However, due to its completely internal nature and its site within the bones of the pelvis, it cannot be immediately viewed during the inspection (Sallustio et al, 2000). Moreover, it is logic to presume that there is a histological picture related to the lymphedema which is comparable to that of other areas: interstitial retention of proteins, tissue inflammation, fatty tissue hypertrophy, fibrosis, progressive pathological condition (Warren et al, 2007). The progressive pathological condition should underlie the disease of the pelvic floor. As above mentioned, pelviperineology is a recent discipline and it is still subject to complex evaluations by many specialists: gynaecologists, urologists, proctologists, sexologists (Jones et al, 2008). The benefits resulting from the treatments of rehabilitation proposed by these specialists indirectly ensure the decongestive action typical for the physical exercise of the other body districts, beyond stimulating the correct recovery of the muscular activity. This should mean that the treatments of rehabilitation of pelvis result in the evident reduction in the edema and the related cohort of symptoms. Indeed, the best way to treat lymphedema and the related disorders seems to be the increase in the force of lymphatic circulation (Swartz et al, 2001). The filtration pressure in the tissue spaces ensures that lymph can move with force and this resulting liquid pressure in the tissue draws the blood from capillaries. The movement of the lymphatic valves provides to lymph the direction from the smaller lymphatic vessels into the lymphatic ducts. The automatic contraction of lymphatic vessels is one of the explanations of the lymphatic circulation and accelerates the formation of the lymph itself. The pressure resulting from the contraction of the adjacent muscles can compress the lymphatic vessels and push the lymphatic circulation towards the valves. It is easy to assume that a pelvic surgery irremediably impairs this fragile balance whereas the rehabilitation offered by the specialists studying the pelvic disorders produces a beneficial decompressing effect on the lymphedema, acting directly on the muscular structure. If this can explain the etiopathogenesis of lymphedema, it is not yet clear why the distribution of this disorder can be so variable. Some peculiar characteristics of the lymphatic vessels in the pelvic area need therefore to be considered. The normal function of the lymphatic vessels is to remove the portion of liquid leaked from the capillaries, which accumulates in the interstice, so that the interstitial pressure can be kept constant (Stachowska-Pietka et al, 2006). The venous capillaries reabsorb 90% of the liquid in the interstice, while the remaining fluid is transported to the blood by the lymphatic vessels in the form of lymph. Under normal conditions, the portion transported to the interstice is the same as that transported in the opposite direction. However, this balance is destroyed in the lymphoadenectomy due to the reduction in the lymph transport capacity. As a result, there is a liquid retention and swelling like in any other body organs after a lymphoadenectomy.

Moreover, the pelvic lymphatic vessels serve to remove macromolecules, such as proteins, from interstice. Unlike other anatomical regions, the particular structure of the pelvis with its parallelepipid shape and semirigid shell, the abundant distribution of venous plexus as well as the tight bond with the intestinal lymphatic tissue make the role of the lymphatic vessels even more specific (Barret et al, 2006). When the proteins diffuse through the arterial capillary wall, they are downgraded by the macrophages, which allow them to come back to the blood circulation through the venous capillary circulation, or are reabsorbed through the lymphatic vessels (Greitz, 2002). During pelvic surgery it is easy to assume that the resulting inflammatory picture will be so widespread that a remarkable number of macrophages will be recruited through the activation of different cell lines and partially contrast the effect of the resulting lymphedema. Moreover, in case of obstructed, abnormal or absent lymphatic system, a lymphatic stasis can occur, leading to retention of proteins and liquid in the interstice. Another element contributes to counteract this effect, namely the close inter-connection with the venous plexus present in the pelvis micro-circulation which acts by mimicking the role of the lymphatic vessels. According to the classical theory, this increase in protein concentration leads to an increase in the tissue colloido–osmotic pressure, which draws liquids into the interstice and causes edema and clinical outbreaks of lymphedema. On the other hand, the intra-abdominal pressure, which ranges from 3 to 5 mm Hg in the postoperative period, contributes to strengthen the effect of lymphedema. Although the intra-abdominal pressure is distributed on the whole cavity, it leads to a higher effect of venous stasis in the operated pelvis, adding to lymphatic pressure. The clinical occurrences of lymphedema occur following the retention of edematogenic liquid in the fatty and subcutaneous tissue. The inflammatory response appears with the liquid retention in the interstitial space. In addition to the inflammation, the slowed lymphatic flow is also associated to an increase in the lipogenesis and fat deposition, to the increase in the activation of fibrocytes and expansion of connective tissue. The patient would progressively develop a subcutaneous hard tissue as a result of the consequent fibrosis in addition to hypertrophy of the fatty tissue. These pathological changes will initially develop as simple swelling, but later on their persistence would lead to a higher state of hardening. Unlike the other regions, the performance of an intra-abdominal surgery, with no contact with the external environment, will never cause the classical signs which are normally visible in another body region. In these terms, it is less difficult to suggest a pelvic lymphedema. Pelvis is a functional unit, therefore, after a surgery (conservative or radical, with or without post-operative treatment); the patients develop pelvic dysfunctions, probably due to lymphedema. We believe that this disorder without an appropriate rehabilitation leads to an inflammation with interstitial liquid retention with high protein concentration, which results in fatty tissue hypertrophy and fibrosis, and develops as a progressive pathological condition. We can therefore agree with the hypothesis that the lymphatic damage leads to pathology of progressive malfunctioning that, if not properly treated, can become chronic within few weeks and result in a severe chronic disease. The pelvic lymphedema can be a difficult condition to be treated and one of those causes with significant morbidity for the patient both from the clinical and psychological points of view. The clinical evidence shows that the lymphatic vessels play a relevant role in the pathology of the pelvic floor and perineum.

5.2 Clinical evidence of pelvic lymphedema

In this pilot study using abdominal MRI we hypothesized that pelvic surgery, regardless of the extra-peritoneal organs, results in the loss of continuity of the pelvic region as key event with the following reduction in fatty extra-peritoneal tissue where the lymph node stations are mostly concentrated; the consequent pelvic lymphadenectomy, should be followed by a pelvic lymphedema (Vannelli et al, 2009). As lymphedema been discovered often by chance and has no reported common elements, it has been difficult to create an experimental model (Savoye-Collet et al, 2008). Here, we attempted to generate a diagnostic model by exploiting the radiological resources available in our laboratory.

Lymphedema results from an alteration of lymphatic vessels as a consequence of malformation (primary) or mechanical damage (secondary) (Warren et al, 2007), consistent with an equal distribution in the upper and lower limbs, neck, scrotum and pubis (Purushotham et al, 2007; Fang et al 2008). Analogously, pelvic lymphedema might be a consequence of mechanical pelvic injury or of the altered lymphatic system caused by such injury. The extra-peritoneal pelvic area is sited between the peritoneum covering the pelvic organs, and the pelvic diaphragm. In the pelvic cavity the peritoneum is separated from the walls which delimit the cavity by the surrounding and supporting fatty extra-peritoneal tissue. Pelvic lymphadenectomy might in itself lead to damaged lymphatic vessels with subsequent pelvic malfunction, within a few weeks post surgery if undiagnosed and untreated, can progress to a chronic pelvic dysfunction. Our post-operative MRIs evidenced injuries involving different pelvic structures and areas, whereas no venous congestion or alteration of lymphatic vessels was detected preoperatively (Table II). Therefore it is of critical importance to investigate the mechanisms of lymphedema in pelvic pathology to limit the consequences of functional abnormalities in patients who undergo conservative surgery. Thus, despite the benefits of surgery, our results support the notion that lymphadenectomy can cause damage of the pelvic lymphatic system as a direct result of surgery. Unlike the common clinical skin signs that characterized all other sites of lymphedema, pelvic lymphedema is "hidden" or silent, with no skin changes or any single symptom manifested (Vannelli et al, 2009). The lack of signs is not surprising, considering that the shell structure of bones of the sacral area provides a structural system capable of containing almost three-fourths of the total volume alterations inside the pelvis without any external manifestations. Moreover, the perineum, which contains no bone structures and thus enables direct and unrestricted internal pelvic communication, is particularly vulnerable to damage caused by lymphadenectomy. This alteration of lymphatic vessels would produce lymphedema or progressive dysfunctional pathology manifesting as muscular deficiency, particularly defective sphincter control. As shown in our MRIs of the bone-tendineal space interposed within a deep plane of the pelvic floor, surgical intervention involving perineal skin "hidden" (Figure 5,6) lymphedema, despite the lymphatic congestion after lymphadenectomy and eventually the conditions for neural and muscular structural malfunction (Handa et al, 2009). In this series, the use of MRI has made it possible to emphasize the pre-operative period in which the presence of the cancer is not associated with any pelvic lymphedema. Moreover, our MRIs showed that pelvic illness alone is accompanied by lymphedema related exclusively to venous congestion, which can be attributed to the neoangiogenesis typically concurrent in these carcinomas. In the post-operative period the effects of lymphadenectomy and opening of the pelvic peritoneum are characterized by specific signs of lymphedema, such as lymphangitis with local fibrosis formation. Actually, the identification of epifascial "lakes" over gluteus muscles in the absence of edema inside of the muscular girdles demonstrates that surgical intervention sets off a domino effect within the pelvic area. The observed venous congestion in areas distant from the interventional area both in patients surgically treated with opening of the extra-peritoneal space and in those without pelvic involvement, further confirms an alteration of pelvic structures following pelvic surgery. Our series of MRIs also identified other common features of lymphedema: accumulation of liquid in adipose tissue or lipedema. The estimate of body fat indicate an average BMI of 29.9 (so called overweight), since reduction of adipose tissue, where lymph nodes are predominantly concentrated, might contribute to the loss of pelvic structural continuity. Moreover, the specific structure of pelvic lymphatics must be considered, since it is ubiquitously and homogenously distributed as a thick net and conveys a "three-dimensional" appearance of volume, unlike the generally single long dimension that characterizes the upper or lower limb lymphatics. Surgery leads not only to the limitation of volume, but also to the involvement of all pelvic structures. To date, lymphedema is frequently undiagnosed even in teaching centers (Schuchhardt C, 1997), and it seems likely that many surgical interventions have not been adequately studied with respect to lymphatic damage and their consequences. Although it could be argued that such studies are not essential when colorectal surgery is only limited to an internal pelvic space, and that any radiological image is only one indictor of type of surgical intervention, we detected signs of venous congestion in all pelvic areas, demonstrating that each surgical procedure implicates involvement of the entire pelvic structure. Thus, it is not the type of surgical intervention that creates favourable conditions for lymphedema, but rather the specific location of the pelvic floor where surgery occurs. The pelvis is a dynamic functional unit endowed with an elastic memory continually responding to changes of: body weight, intra-abdominal pressure due to increased loads caused by chronic conditions, and by the natural events of pregnancy and delivery. Elastic memory of the pelvis contributes in inhibiting the onset of lymphedema. However, surgical disruption of this functional unit, in particular impairment of the pelvic memory capability is exceeded can lead to hides lymphedema. Overall this can be the key factor in explaining pelvic dysfunction.

6. Conclusion

Clinical evidence obtained by MRI in our pilot study indicates that lymphatic vessels play a significant role in surgeries that involve perineum and the pelvic floor (Boekhuis et al, 2009; Campisi, 1991). This pilot study could answer the question ''how does pelvic lymphedema occur?''. During surgery the primary cause responsible for the damage should be detected otherwise if, not promptly treated, it can result in a chronic disease. However a better understanding of pelvic lymphedema could be the key to improving therapeutic strategies, including the routine use of biofeedback re-education of the pelvic floor, for functional abnormalities after pelvic surgery (Striefel & Glazer, 2008).

7. Acknowledgments

The authors thank Dr Patrizia Gasparini who helped write and revise the paper and Mrs. Roberta Aceto for her assistance with data collection.

8. References

Andrade, M. & Jacomo, A. (2007). Anatomy of the human lymphatic system. *Cancer Treatment and Research*, Vol.135, (January 2007), pp. 55–77, ISSN 0927-3042

Antolak, Jr SJ.; Hough, D.M.; Pawlina, W. & Spinner, R.J. (2002). Anatomical basis of chronic pelvis pain syndrome: The ischial spine and pudendal nerve entrapment. *Medical Hypotheses* Vol.59, N. 3, (September 2002), pp. 349–53, ISSN 0306-9877

Aström KG.; Abdsaleh S.; Brenning GC. & Ahlström KH. (2001). MR imaging of primary, secondary, and mixed forms of lymphedema. *Acta Radiologica* Vol.42, N.2, (July 2001), pp. 409-16, ISSN 0365-5954

Bai, SW.; Huh, EH.; Jung, da J.; Park, JH.; Rha, KH.; Kim, SK. & Park, KH. (2006). Urinary tract injuries during pelvic surgery: incidence rates and predisposing factors. *International Urogynecology Journal and Pelvic Floor Dysfunction* Vol.17, N.4, (June 2006), pp. 360-4, ISSN 1433-3023

Barrett, T.; Choyke, PL. & Kobayashi, H. (2006). Imaging of the lymphatic system: new horizons. *Contrast Media & Molecular Imaging*, Vol.1, N.6, (Nov-Dec 2006), pp. 230-45 ISSN 1555-4317

Blackledge, G. (2003). Cancer Drugs: The next ten years. *European Journal of Cancer*, Vol. 39, No. 3, (February 2003), pp. 273, ISSN: 0959-8049

Breyer, BN.; Greene, KL.; Dall'Era, MA.; Davies, BJ. & Kane, CJ. (2008). Pelvic lymphadenectomy in prostate cancer. *Prostate Cancer and Prostatic Diseases*, Vol.11, N.4, (May 2008), pp. 320-4, ISSN 1365- 7852

Broekhuis, SR.; Kluivers, KB.; Hendriks, JC.; Vierhout, ME.; Barentsz, JO. & Fütterer JJ. (2009). Dynamic magnetic resonance imaging: reliability of anatomical landmarks and reference lines used to assess pelvic organ prolapse. *International Urogynecology Journal and Pelvic Floor Dysfunction*, Vol.20, N.2, (February 2009), pp. 141-8, ISSN 1433-3023

Brown, SR. & Seow-Choen, F. (2000). Preservation of rectal function after low anterior resection with formation of a neorectum. *Seminars in Surgical Oncology*, Vol.19, N.4, (December 2000), pp. 376-85, ISSN 1098-2388

Campisi, C. (1991). A rational approach to the management of lymphedema. *Lymphology*, Vol.24, N.2, (June 1991), pp. 48-53, ISSN 0024-7766

Clarke, AC.; (1962) Hazards of prophecy :The failure of imagination in Profiles of the Future, Harper & Row, ISBN 0-445-04061-0, New York

Corton, MM. (2005). Anatomy of the pelvis: how the pelvis is built for support. *Clinical Obstetrics and Gynecology*, Vol.48, N.3, (September 2005), pp. 611-26, ISSN 1532-5520

Delfaut, EM.; Beltran, J.; Johnson, G.; Rousseau, J.; Marchandise, X. & Cotton, A. (1999). Fat suppression in MR imaging: techniques and pitfalls. *Radiographics*, Vol.19, N.2, (Mar-Apr 1999), pp. 373-82, ISSN 1527-1323

Desnoo, L. & Faithfull, S. (2006). A qualitative study of anterior resection syndrome: the experiences of cancer survivors who have undergone resection surgery. *European Journal of Cancer Care (Engl)*, Vol.15, N.3, (July 2006), pp. 244-51, ISSN 1365-2354

Devroede, G. (1999). Front and rear: the pelvic floor is an integrated functional structure. *Medical Hypotheses*, Vol.52, N.2, (February 1999), pp. 147-53, ISSN 0306-9877

Ebisu, T.; Naruse, S.; Horikawa, Y.; Ueda, S.; Tanaka, C.; Uto, M.; Umeda, M. & Higuchi, T. (1993). Discrimination between different types of white matter edema with diffusion-weighted MR imaging. *Journal of Magnetic Resonance Imaging*, Vol.3, N.6, (Nov-Dec 1993), pp. 863-8, ISSN 1053-1807

Fang, Y.; He, Y. & Liu, Z. (2008). Negative pressure in pharyngo-oral cavity can treat lymphedema and related disorders. *Medical Hypotheses*, Vol.70, N.4, (October 2008), pp.886-7, ISSN 0306-9877

Greco, P.; Andreola, S.; Magro, G.; Belli, F.; Giannone, G.; Gallino, GF. & Leo, E. (2006). Potential pathological understaging of pT3 rectal cancer with less than 26 lymph nodes recovered: a prospective study based on a resampling of 50 rectal specimens. *Virchows Archives*, Vol.449, N.6, (December 2006), pp. 647-51, ISSN 1432-2307

Greitz D. (2002). On the active vascular absorption of plasma proteins from tissue: Rethinking the role of the lymphatic system. *Medical Hypotheses*, Vol.59, N.6, (December 2002), pp. 696–702, ISSN 0306-9877

Gummere, RM. (1917-25). 3 vols. Volume I. Epistle LXIV, In: *Lucius Annaeus Seneca. Moral Epistles. Translated by Richard M. Gummere*. The Loeb Classical Library, pp. 117, Cambridge, Mass.: Harvard UP, Retrived from <http://www.stoics.com/seneca_epistles_book_1.html>

Handa, VL.; Lockhart, ME.; Kenton, KS.; Bradley, CS.; Fielding, JR.; Cundiff, GW.; Salomon, CG.; Hakim, C.; Ye, W. & Richter, HE. (2009). Magnetic resonance assessment of pelvic anatomy and pelvic floor disorders after childbirth. *International Urogynecology Journal of Pelvic Floor Dysfunction*, Vol.20, N.2, (February 2009), pp. 133-9, ISSN 1433-3023

Jones, GL.; Radley, SC.; Lumb, J. & Jha, S. (2008). Electronic pelvic floor symptoms assessment: Tests of data quality of ePAQ-PF. *International Urogynecology Journal of Pelvic Floor Dysfunction*, Vol.19, N.10, (October 2008), pp. 1337-47, ISSN 1433-3023

Kakodkar, R.; Gupta, S. & Nundy, S. (2006). Low anterior resection with total mesorectal excision for rectal cancer: functional assessment and factor affecting outcome. *Colorectal Disease,*; Vol.8, N.8, (October 2006), pp. 650-6, ISSN 1463-1318

Leo, E.; Belli, F.; Miceli, R.; Mariani, L.; Gallino, G.; Battaglia, L.; Vannelli, A. & Andreola, S. (2009). Distal clearance margin of 1 cm or less: a safe distance in lower rectum cancer surgery. *International Journal of Colorectal Diseases*, Vol.24, N.3, (March 2009), pp. 317-22, ISSN 1432-1262

Lohrmann, C.; Foeldi, E. & Langer, M. (2009). MR imaging of the lymphatic system in patients with lipedema and lipo-lymphedema: *Microvascular Research*, Vol.77, N.3, (May 2009), pp. 335-9, ISSN 0026-2862

Mills, RD.; Fleischmann, A. & Studer, UE. (2007). Radical cystectomy with an extended pelvic lymphadenectomy: rationale and results. *Surgical Oncology Clinics of North* America, Vol.16, N.1, (January 2007), pp. 233-45, ISSN: 1055-3207

Ortiz, H. & Armendariz P. (1996). Anterior resection: do the patients perceive any clinical benefit? *International Journal of Colorectal Diseases*, Vol.11, N.4, (xxx 1996), pp. 191-5. ISSN 1432-1262

Peters, K.; Girdler, B.; Carrico, D.; Ibrahim, I. & Diokno, A. (2008). Painful bladder syndrome/interstitial cystitis and vulvodynia: A clinical correlation. *International Urogynecology Journal of Pelvic Floor Dysfunction*, Vol.19, N.5, (May 2008), pp. 665-9 ISSN 1433-3023

Purushotham, AD.; Bennett Britton, TM.; Klevesath, MB.; Chou, P.; Agbaje, OF. & Duffy, SW. (2007). Lymph node status and breast cancer-related lymphedema. *Annal of Surgery*, Vol.246, N.1, (July 2007), pp. 42-5, ISSN 1528-1140

Sallustio, G.; Giangregorio, C.; Cannas, L.; Vricella, D.; Celi, G. & Rinaldi, P. (2000), Lymphatic system: Morphofunctional considerations. *Rays*, Vol.25, N.4 (Oct-Dec 2000), pp. 419-27, ISSN 0390-7740

Savoye-Collet, C.; Koning, E.; & Dacher, JN. (2008). Radiologic evaluation of pelvic floor disorders. *Gastroenterology Clinics of North America*, Vol.37, N.3, (September 2008), pp. 553-67, ISSN 0889-8553

Schuchhardt, C. (1997). Lymphedema. An easy diagnosis--but frequently missed. *Fortschritte der Medizin*, Vol. 20, N.115, (August 1997), pp. 24, 27-31, ISSN 0946-5634

Selke, B.; Durand, I.; Marissal, JP.; Chevalier, D. & Lebrun, T. (2003). Cost of colorectal cancer in France in 1999. *Gastroentérologie Clinique et Biologique,* Vol.27, N.1, (January 2003), pp. 22-7, ISSN 0399-8320

Stachowska-Pietka, J.; Waniewski, J.; Flessner, MF. & Lindholm, B. (2006). Distributed model of peritoneal fluid absorption. *American Journal of Physiology - Heart and Circulatory Physiology*, Vol.291, N.4, (October 2006), pp. 1862-74, ISSN 0363-6135

Striefel, S. & Glazer, HI. (2008). A proposed set of ethical practice guidelines in the assessment and treatment of pelvic floor disorders. *Applied Psychophysiology and Biofeedback,* Vol.33, N.4, (December 2008), pp. 181-93, ISSN 1573-3270

Swartz, MA. (2001). The physiology of the lymphatic system. *Advanced Drug Delivery Reviews,* Vol.23, N.50(1-2), (August 2001), pp. 3-20, ISSN 0169-409X

Taneja, C. & Cady, B. (2005). Decreasing role of lymphatic system surgery in surgical oncology. *Journal of Surgical Oncology,* Vol.1, N.89(2), (February 2005), pp. 61-6, ISSN 1096-9098

Thorat, MA. (2006). Are there distinct lymphatic flow patterns in the breast? *Medical Hypotheses,* Vol.66, N.5, (January 2006), pp. 1040-1, ISSN 0306-9877

Van der Putte, SC. (2005). The development of the perineum in the human. A comprehensive histological study with a special reference to the role of the stromal components. *Advances in Anatomy, Embryology, and Cell Biology,* Vol.177, (2005), pp. 1-131, ISSN 0301-5556

Vannelli, A.; Battaglia, L.; Poiasina, E. & Leo E. Pelvic lymphedema: Truth or fiction? *Medical Hypotheses,* Vol.72, N.3, (March 2009), pp. 267-70, ISSN 0306-9877

Vignes, S. & Trévidic, P. (2005). Lymphedema of male external genitalia: a retrospective study of 33 cases. *Annales de dermatologie et de venereologie,* Vol.132, N.1, (January 2005), pp. 21-5, ISSN 0151-9638

Warren, AG.; Brorson, H.; Borud, LJ. & Slavin, SA. (2007).Lymphedema - a comprehensive review. *Annals of Plastic Surgery,* Vol.59, N.4, (October 2007), pp. 464-72, ISSN 1536-3708

Wilting, J.; Papoutsim, M. & Becker, J. (2004). The lymphatic vascular system: Secondary or primary? *Lymphology,* Vol.37, N.3, (September 2004), pp. 98-106, ISSN 0024-7766

Winawer, S. (2007) Colorectal cancer screening, In: World Gastroenterology Organisation/International Digestive Cancer Alliance Practice Guidelines, date of access 2011, available from:
http://www.worldgastroenterology.org/assets/downloads/en/pdf/guidelines/06_colorectal_cancer_screening.pdf

Witte CL. (2002) Quality of life. *Lymphology*, Vol.35, N.2 (June 2002), pp. 44-5 ISSN 0024-7766
Zermann, DH.; Ishigooka, M.; Doggweiler-Wiygul, R.; Schubert, J. & Schmidt, RA. (2001). The male chronic pelvic pain syndrome. *World Journal of Urology*, Vol.19, N.3, June 2001), pp. 173-9, ISSN 1433-8726